W9-CLA-944

WITHDRAWN
No longer the property of the
Boston Public Library.
Sale of this material benefits the Library.

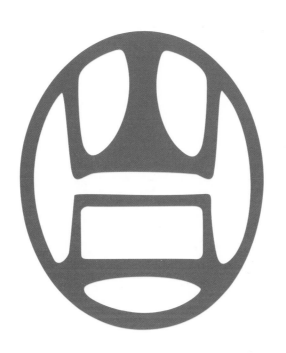

billy yamaguchi
feng shui beauty

billy yamaguchi
feng shui beauty

bringing the ancient
principles of balance and
harmony to your hair,
makeup and personal style

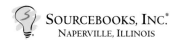
SOURCEBOOKS, INC.®
NAPERVILLE, ILLINOIS

Copyright © 2004 by Billy Yamaguchi

Cover and internal design © 2004 by Sourcebooks, Inc.

Cover photos © Toshihiko Sawajiri and Getty Images

Internal model photos © Toshihiko Sawajiri

Sourcebooks and the colophon are registered trademarks of Sourcebooks, Inc.

All rights reserved. No part of this book may be reproduced in any form or by any electronic or mechanical means including information storage and retrieval systems—except in the case of brief quotations embodied in critical articles or reviews—without permission in writing from its publisher, Sourcebooks, Inc.

Published by Sourcebooks, Inc.

P.O. Box 4410, Naperville, Illinois 60567-4410

(630) 961-3900

FAX: (630) 961-2168

www.sourcebooks.com

Library of Congress Cataloging-in-Publication Data

Yamaguchi, Billy.
  Billy Yamaguchi feng shui beauty / by Billy Yamaguchi.
    p. cm.
  ISBN 1-4022-0323-3 (alk. paper)
  1. Hairstyles. 2. Beauty culture. 3. Feng shui. 1. Title.

TT972.Y33 2004
646.7'042—dc22
        2004016059

Printed and bound in the United States of America

QW   10 9 8 7 6 5 4 3 2 1

To Melissa, Seiji, Nobu, and the spirit of my
Obaachan Kimi Yamaguchi and Ojiichan Kanzo Yamaguchi.

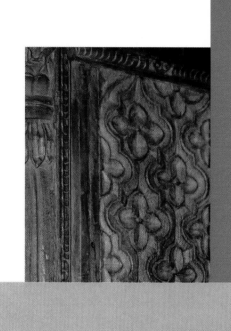
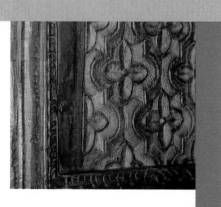

Table of Contents

Acknowledgments

As many authors have said before me, writing a book is no solitary feat. I would like to thank and acknowledge the following people for their considerable contributions to me, to my work, and to this book:

The gracious clients who over many years have participated in the growth and testing of the thoughts, ideas, and techniques of Feng Shui beauty. They have been supportive and loyal.

My mentors in the industry: Hans Wolf, Eric Knudsen, Jerry Gordon, Horst Rechelbacher, Yosh Toya, and Don Shaw. They were my inspiration and their advice has been invaluable.

George Broder, Heinz Bieler, Bobby Peels, the Schwarzkopf family, the Shannon family, and all our distributors for their support and the opportunity for growth.

Lillian Too, one of the great scholars and authors of Feng Shui, taught both Melissa and me.

Phil Jackson, kindred spirit and close friend on the journey. His friendship has given me a unique sense of perspective and encouraged me to appreciate both the forest and the trees.

Dominique Raccah and Deb Werksman, my publisher and my editor at Sourcebooks. The book was waiting for them.

Victoria Brown, my publicist at Sourcebooks, for her continuing hard work and dedication.

To all of the Yamaguchi team whose support has never wavered as they have lived our dream each day.

To Toni Hill, our corporate color director, who is an integral part of our company. She has been a worthy participant in this journey of Feng Shui and contributed greatly to this book.

Cory Chambers, who has always supported me and contributed many illustrations to this book. He has attended to many details, enabling me to be creative.

If creating a book is like birthing a baby, Patricia Shepherd and Doug Chambers were the midwives. Working together, we took the dream of this concept and breathed life into it. Without them, I can honestly say there would be no book. Patricia has coached me, challenged me to develop and share my gifts, trained me to speak in public, and introduced me to a myriad of ideas. For what she has provided me, both personally and professionally, no thanks could ever be enough.

All of the others, too numerous to name, who have supported, coached, and taught me along the way.

To my parents, Taeko and John, with much love and gratitude.

Melissa Chambers Yamaguchi, my wife, my inspiration, and the visionary who pushed me out of my box and made me everything that I am today. Melissa introduced me to Feng Shui, and brings its timeless wisdom and depth into every aspect of our life and our family. Her influence and contribution to this book were invaluable. Without her and our beautiful children, Seiji and Nobu, all the rest would mean nothing.

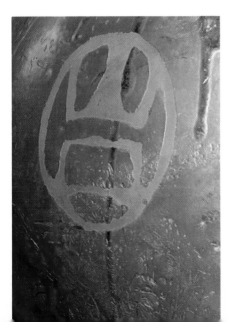

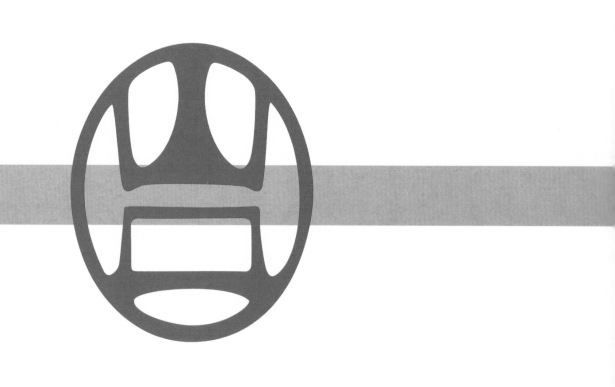

billy yamaguchi
feng shui beauty

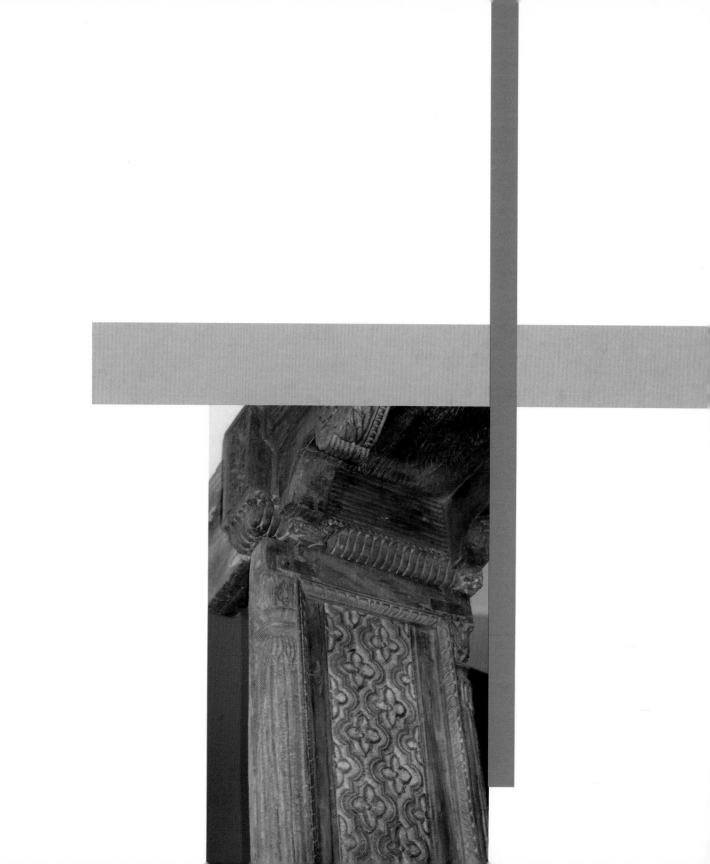

1 Introduction to Feng Shui Beauty

Some of my happiest memories are from my times as a small child in Fujisawa in the Kamakura area of Japan. My grandfather Kanzo Yamaguchi took me on long walks to Kamakura and to Enoshima Island; he shared stories of his past and taught me how to see the beauty in my environment. As I grew older, he took me to the local temples where the wooden Tori gates served as a reminder that we were entering a sacred area. I can still vividly remember my fascination with the movement of the koi fish, the placement of the rocks, the sound of the chimes, and the aromatic incense that permeated the gardens. Ojiichan (Grandfather) taught me to listen to the silence so that I might hear the harmony of the world. Although many people surrounded us, I remember the serenity of these excursions as if my grandfather and I were the only ones on the island. I did not understand this special feeling at the time...this energy...this Chi.

When I began my career as a hairstylist, I was content to hone my technical skills. I've always been passionate about my work; nevertheless, I felt that something was lacking although by most standards I was successful early in my career. When my wife, Melissa, began the study of Feng Shui, she would share with me its ancient philosophy as related to design. I began a journey of discovery through our exchanges about Feng Shui; I learned about the art of placement used in architecture, interior design, and gardens to create the flow of Chi. Chi is commonly translated as energy; however, Chi moves and flows much like water. In popular culture, Feng Shui is most commonly associated with the placement of objects, yet I felt that it had wider application. For years I had been telling my clients to honor themselves as a temple and to be mindful of what they put in or on their temple. With this in mind and looking at the individual as a temple, my thought was that the first step in creating good Chi must begin with the self. I began my study of Feng Shui roughly ten years ago and have continued my quest for providing the most accurate roadmap to understanding individual energy.

Feng Shui is a fascinating and complex discipline. Although generally recognized as a guide for the proper energy manipulation of the home and garden, Feng Shui is much more. Feng Shui is a guide to understanding individual energies, both fixed and fluctuating. The energy elements with which one is born may not change; however, due to life's experiences and the development of one's personality, other energy elements will change. These fluctuating energy elements are what I am most interested in.

Feng Shui masters deal with the energy of fixed objects like furniture, live objects like trees and gardens, and with the factual data of individuals for a more personal energy reading. These energy readings and understandings cannot be compared to the volatile, changing, electric energy I work with daily: that of the human spirit.

I see guests who are undergoing terrific change in their lives. Women who have survived cancer; men who just lost their jobs; women who have discovered they're pregnant for the first time; young adults accepted to the college of their choice; guests who have just lost a loved one. You can imagine the tremendous energy changes that I deal with visit to visit. I discovered that these life changes greatly affect how the guest sees herself. That same old haircut and color may not work appointment after appointment. Yet, isn't that what a lot of hairstylists do? Give the guest the same old cut/color out of habit? I know I did for years. You see, your hair changes, your fashion sense changes, your skin and nails change and this is where I come in.

To learn more about self or the individual, I studied the five elements in Feng Shui. All five elements, Fire, Earth, Metal, Water, and Wood, are present in everyone. At any given time, however, two elements will be more dominant depending on the life stages and experiences of the individual. The five elements are each associated with distinct characteristics, colors, and shapes. I began the study, adaptation, and application of Feng Shui to my lifestyle and to the world of beauty.

I am a people watcher by nature; in a very real sense, this study of people has been my college education. I listen to and study my clients as well as the people around me. I wanted to discover what makes an individual have a presence that causes others to notice and to remember. This intangible quality in an individual seems to be an embodiment of good energy, or Chi. This individual has power. For these individuals, there seems to be a harmony between their physical presence and their personality. Was this something learned or inherent in individuals? Was there a connection between self-knowledge and self-expression? As a designer of beauty, could I create a style for the individual that would reflect "who she really is"—her essence—and thus release her power (Chi)?

Although I could observe the outside of the individual, I needed a method of understanding more about how the individual saw herself. With this in mind, I revisited the five elements, considering these five elements as a basis to identify or classify an individual. Utilizing a questionnaire containing the characteristics and colors of the five elements, designers could identify or classify the two colors that were most predominant. The Feng Shui Consultation was created using this method. The Feng Shui Consultation is the starting point for all Feng Shui services. In this book, I have expanded the Consultation which can be found in chapters three though five.

I have adapted the art and principles of Feng Shui to all aspects of beauty: cutting, color, makeup, nails, massage, and exercise. When the Eastern principles of Feng Shui are combined with a Western holistic approach, the beauty industry is elevated to a new level. It is my belief that Feng Shui will revolutionize the beauty industry.

In order to explain our approach, we've used traditional Feng Shui terminology, but redefined or redesigned them as pertaining to the beauty industry. I have redesigned the geomancer's compass, called a luo pan (pronounced "low pan"), as a tool to enhance, harmonize, or balance the dominant element. This tool is utilized after the dominant element has been identified. In Chapter 5, you will determine where you belong on the element barometer. You can then decide to enhance, harmonize, or balance.

Some people are curious and sometimes skeptical about the adaptation of Feng Shui to the beauty industry. Some have called Feng Shui a fad; however, I know of no fad that has been in existence for almost four thousand years. In my salons, our use of this Feng Shui approach invites more expression from the clients about who they are and offers a framework for explaining the need to honor themselves or their temple. For me, the study of Feng Shui has become a lifestyle. My study of Feng Shui has helped me to realize that I will forever be a student of Feng Shui and never a master, for this process is a never-ending course of discovery. My family and I have adapted this discipline and science to all aspects of our life. It has brought order and beauty to our universe.

So, for you, this book is a roadmap to understanding the energy of the individual according to the rules of Feng Shui and my professional experiences. My intention is for you to discover who you are, who you want to be, and then to be able to have that expression shine through. And before you ask, "But, isn't it only a cut?" remember the last time you received a cut, color, makeup application, or new outfit, looked in the mirror and thought, "Wow! I look great!"

Every experience should be so wonderful. I aim to help you achieve it.

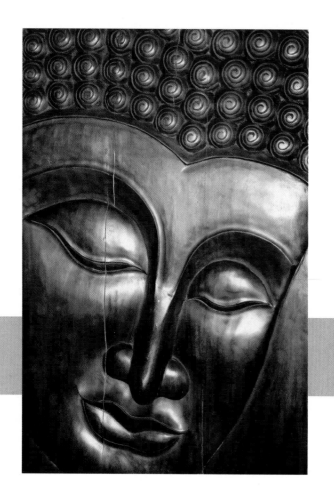

2 Feng Shui

The Chinese art of utilizing the forces of the universe to organize lives is generally thought to have originated over seven thousand years ago. From this ancient practice, Feng Shui originated in the mountains of China over thirty-five hundred years ago and has its roots in China's agrarian tradition. The farmers' battle to survive, and eventually to prosper, hinged on a grasp of nature's changes and its forces and of the earth's energies. The focus on the movement of wind and water (the literal meaning of Feng Shui) was the basis of Feng Shui. The Taoist masters greatly respected nature and believed that the study and understanding of nature was the answer to many of life's questions. The relationship between man and these unseen forces of nature were observed, studied, recorded, and respected.

The early mandarins saw rural farmers as the backbone of society. The farmers represented stability and brought balance to society. The study of the earth and its relationship to the provisions of the farmer were greatly respected. Studies of the growth of crops in every conceivable direction were recorded. From these studies came an understanding of the energies emitted from the earth. Observing the stars and recording events in the night skies was another method of study. Nightly practice of recording the stars led to the ability to predict both solar and lunar eclipses with considerable accuracy. This knowledge was encoded into the calendar system and gave tremendous weight to the energy descending from heaven.

Feng Shui is derived from the teachings of the *I Ching*, which dates back to legendary antiquity. The mother of all Chinese philosophy, science, beliefs, and cultural history, the *I Ching* greatly influenced Chinese scholars as well as both branches of Chinese philosophy, Confucianism and Taoism. It instructed emperors, priests, scholars, and military leaders on the advisability of anything from waging war to travel. It also served as a guidepost for understanding human traits, fortune, health, romance, and other concerns.

The *I Ching* represents the principle of never-changing and ever-changing. The order of the seasons of the year—winter, spring, summer, and fall—never change; the actual seasons year to year do change. This year's summer wasn't exactly like last year's and yet, they were both classified as summer. You were born and were christened, perhaps with the name Mary. You are still Mary today, yet you are physically, emotionally, and mentally different than you were when you were born. Your existence is never-changing, but you are ever-changing and evolving with life's experiences. Life is never frozen in any one state. The process that links the state of man to that of the universe is known as Tao.

Tao is a thread that serves to connect man with the universe. It integrates Chinese custom and wisdom, astrology, herbal medicine, and Feng Shui to achieve happiness.

Tao was originally referred to as The Way or The Path. The Taoist ideal is to lead a simple, spontaneous, and meditative life close to nature. The yearning for a life in harmony with nature was the Taoist principle. Taoism states that man should mirror nature, following the same laws as nature; in doing so, he must understand his relationship to nature by studying interacting opposites. Tao represents the wholeness of the universe. Opposites continually spawn each other, creating a whole, or Tao. The circular symbol of Taoism is the Tai-Chi, epitomizing Yin/Yang. The Taoist search for knowledge of nature led many to search for answers in various sciences.

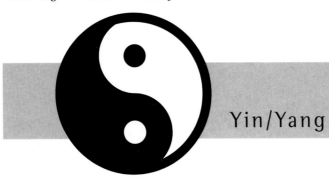

Yin/Yang

Out of Tao came Yin and Yang. Yin and Yang are the two primordial forces that govern the universe. They are complementary opposites that make up all aspects of life and matter. The Yin and Yang essence is as follows: the universe is run by a single principle, the Tao. This principle is divided into two opposite or opposing principles, Yin and Yang. Under Yang are the principles of the sun, heat, light, maleness, hardness, noise, the outdoors, dominance, and heaven, while Yin principles are the moon, cold, darkness, female, softness, quiet, indoors, submission, and earth. Each opposite produces the other and occurs constantly and cyclically. One is neither dominant nor submissive to the other eternally. All conditions are subject to change. All events have within them the beginnings of their opposite state: sickness has potential for health, wealth that of poverty, and so on. No occurrence is completely without its opposite counter.

Without the concept of one, the other would not exist. The opposites are connected in a never-ending cycle of interaction and interdependence. Each of us has characteristics of both Yin and Yang. At one point, one principle may be more evident than the other. Should you suffer from depression, insist on wearing black, and become introverted, you would be displaying principles of Yin. Were you, on the other hand, extremely charismatic, wearing bright, eye-catching colors, and gregarious in personality, you would be considered Yang. The symbol serves to remind us that just when we think we know all there is to know about someone or something, there is another side to consider. Nothing is all black or white (Yin or Yang), but always changing. Yin is the power of nurturing—the softer side, while Yang is the directive, forceful activity side. The Yin/Yang theory is a model of the constant process of change, the transformation of energy. Nothing and no one is entirely Yin or entirely Yang.

All matter has vibration: the Hindus recognize it as Prana, the Hebrews call it Ruach, the Greeks call it Pneuma, the Japanese call it Ki, and the Chinese call it Chi. According to Feng Shui, the force that links man and his surroundings is called Chi. There are different types of Chi: that which circulates in the earth, that which flows in the atmosphere, and that which stirs within our physical bodies. Each of us has Chi. Chi moves our bodies. The characteristics and the manner in which Chi moves in each of us are different. The way Chi fills our bodies determines how we affect others in our environment and in our world.

Chi circulates within the earth, constantly moving, always pulsating. Chi roughly translates as the life force or cosmic breath which pervades all of life. Chi is the basic form of energy that permeates the material universe. All energy and even the finest matter have Chi. It is the energy that links the mind to the heart to the body to our surrounding environment and world. Chi is what brings life and is what distinguishes between living and dead matter. Chi both influences and is influenced; therefore, it is in a constant state of flux. There are two types of energy: negative, or Sha Chi, which can be visualized as bullets; and positive, or Sheng Chi, which can be visualized as a vibrant, fluid arch like the wave of the ocean. When Sheng Chi exists between you and those around you, effortless, comfortable feelings are present.

Everything in your environment affects you and your Chi: the weather, the landscape, the building you are in, your car, someone else's perfume, the sun, the food you eat, etc. Chi is the energy flowing from the hairstylist's arm down to the scissors; it is the energy flowing in the acupuncture meridians; it brings forth fertile crops. In Chinese martial arts, Chi is the controlled power that allows the body to kick. Chi naturally flows in a meandering course. When it flows gently, abundance follows. When it becomes stagnant, life dries up. When it rushes rapidly, it becomes destructive. So it is with the Chi in us: when we slow down and allow our energy to flow gently, we become successful. When we become stagnant or do not aspire to grow and to learn, our life seems boring and meaningless. When we rush rapidly headlong through life, we become stressed and our actions become destructive to our health, goals, and success. The ideal situation for Feng Shui is to harness the positive Chi so that it flows with abundance and is optimized.

As the energy that circulates in our bodies, Chi both moves and motivates us. It sets our personalities and individual movements as well as determines our destiny and potential. Once we are able to acknowledge and understand our Chi and the energy around us, we can use this knowledge to influence our actions and surroundings.

Yin and Yang join in a productive and harmonious union and give birth to the five elements. These manifestations of Chi are the powers or essences of all matter, symbolized by Fire, Earth, Metal, Water, and Wood. These elements are considered the basic building blocks of everything physical on the planet. Feng Shui observes that human beings are made up of all five elements. In Chinese thought, each of these essences is associated with specific colors, matter, moods, tastes, organs of the body, and variations of time and space. Each element has its own Chi characteristic. The whole universe is in a state of constant flux with everything interrelated and interdependent for existence in its own duality—this is called a thermodynamic process. That process is identified in Feng Shui in three cycles labeled productive, exhaustive, and destructive.

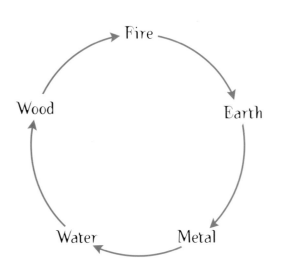

The productive sequence for the elements is as follows: Fire warms Earth, Earth supplements Metal, Metal condenses into Water, Water nourishes Wood, and Wood feeds Fire. This is the harmonizing sequence that adds to the elements.

Productive sequence

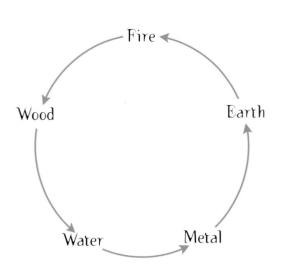

The exhaustive sequence is as follows: Fire overtakes Wood, Wood absorbs Water, Water rusts Metal, Metal depletes Earth, and Earth stops Fire. This is the harmonizing sequence that diminishes the elements.

Exhaustive sequence

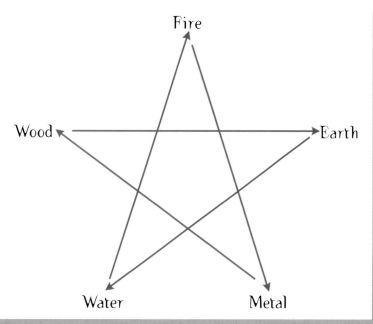

Fire

Wood

Earth

Water

Metal

The destructive sequence is in this order: Fire melts Metal, Metal cuts Wood, Wood robs Earth, Earth absorbs Water, and Water puts out Fire. We refer to this sequence as balancing.

Destructive sequence

Although people have qualities of each element, two will normally dominate at any give time. In general, Fire people are often leaders and crave attention. Earth people are supportive and loyal. Metal people are dogmatic and resolute. Water people are diplomatic and intuitive. Wood people are energetic and social. Keep in mind that everything is either more Yin or more Yang in relation to other things. Everything seeks a state of balance. In all beings and in all matter, the Yin and Yang balance is constantly changing. Your mood and the way you react to events depend on whether you feel more Yin or Yang at a particular time. (Chapter 5, Yin/Yang Energy, shows the Yin and Yang of each element and has a checklist so you can determine whether you are Yin or Yang in relation to your elements.)

Throughout the ages, man has relied upon the arrangement of the stars, sun, and moon in the universe to serve as his compass. This reliance upon the power of the heavens and the energy of the universe has been found in all cultures. People of all civilizations, both present and past, have been keenly attuned to their connection to the energy of the universe and how it interacted with their life and the life forces around them.

For example, in the United States the pioneer farmers knew that seeds were affected by planting at certain cycles of the moon and that animals were affected by these forces from conception to birth to slaughter. Farmers would breed and even slaughter their animals according to phases of the moon. (In our agrarian background, our farmers utilized the cycles of the moon for planting and harvesting, and believed that birth was more liable to occur during certain cycles of the moon.) Early settlers used the almanac as a source for reading the cycles of the moon and for understanding the energies that surrounded them. In our modern commercial world, many have lost the primal connection to the energy of the universe and fail to recognize it as the life force that sustains, influences, and provides a harmonious and balanced relationship within ourselves, others, and our universe.

We are all affected by energy. We have all walked into a home for the first time and either felt totally comfortable or ill at ease. We have met someone for the first time and felt as though we had known that person forever. The energy was good; we connected. We have also walked into a room and felt that something was wrong or met someone and felt uncomfortable—sometimes we call this instinct, but it is really our subconscious perception of the negative energy in the room.

The complete understanding of Feng Shui takes time and dedication. The study of the *I Ching* takes scholars years of focus on its layers of meaning and nuances. The acceptance of Taoist practices is somewhat easy: the realization of man's relationship to nature merely requires attention and commitment. The Yin Yang theory is digestible in its infancy; however, once one takes on the deeper meaning as it relates to the elements, open-minded learning must be the guide. To grasp fully and feel Chi, one must abandon the Western teaching of the need for hardcore evidence. The five elements and all they offer are understandable. Remembering to apply the rules of the five elements to everything in your environment and in you takes dedication. The discipline of Feng Shui is not simplistic and cannot be fully grasped in a few brief hours of reading. Its rules, principles, and time-tested systems require devoted and committed study for a complete appreciation of its rich nuances.

In exchange for deeper examination into the fascinating study of Feng Shui, we can gain a heightened awareness of both the world around us and our relationship to the world. With this awareness comes a sense of empowerment: tools to impact our lives are within our reach.

Even if you are not interested in undertaking an in-depth study of Feng Shui, a grasp of the core concepts as they relate to the individual described in this book can still have a meaningful impact on your life. By digesting the notion that all energy is interconnected, that your energy is affected by the things around you, and that you can use this relationship to influence your life, you will realize the powerful role you can play in directing the story of your life. By recognizing the elements' roles in our personalities and lifestyles, you can better understand your likes and dislikes, your hopes and fears, and your needs. Moreover, an understanding of the elements can give you novel insight into how to better interact with people and how to predict what will resonate with those with whom you interact and what will cause them to recoil.

For those of you that do wish to pursue a study of Feng Shui, there are endless resources. Among the fine authors in this field is Lillian Too. Ms. Too is the most prolific writer on Feng Shui, and writes in an approachable, practical style.

Should you continue your study of Feng Shui, or in the event you've already read one or more books about Feng Shui or even attended a lecture on the topic, you'll find that there are several disciplines and varying interpretations. While each has its merits and offers valuable insights, I often notice confusion when people try to reconcile the differences between these varying schools of thought. Instead of viewing the varying schools as being at odds, I prefer to consider them as alternative heartfelt interpretations of one phenomenon. I recall the old tale about the three blind men separately led to an elephant and asked to describe the elephant. The first took its trunk in his hands and described the elephant as being like a snake. The second, after running his hands over the elephant's leg, likened the elephant to a tree. The third, with only its tail within his grasp, confidently described the elephant as being like a rope. Each interpretation was accurate in terms of what details were being examined.

Our adaptation of Feng Shui is limited and knowingly ignores some of the concepts that are important to a broader understanding of the discipline. We'll concentrate on three fundamental Feng Shui principals: Yin/Yang, the five elements, and Chi. We've focused on the energy between beauty stylist and as well as the the influence of people in your life and the energy between you and these people.

I have taken my respect for Feng Shui and adapted it to my love for the beauty industry. My Yamaguchi Feng Shui Beauty will enable you to determine the best look for you. Not the best look for your neighbor, for the latest, hottest celebrity, or for the you of ten years ago—the best look for the you of today. Who you are now, what describes your life now, and what your tastes are should determine the look you receive.

The only request I have of you is that you enter this system with an open mind and an honest view. Let's begin.

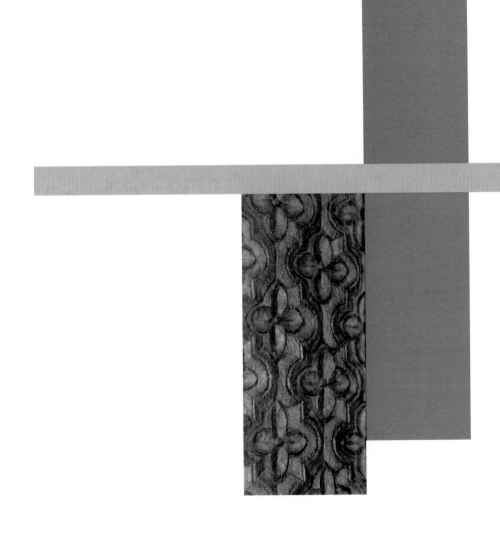

3 It's All About You!

So far, you've read an introduction to Feng Shui and learned about how we created our approach. Now it is time to look inward; for this chapter, it is all about you.

This chapter will take you through an exercise that will be very similar to the dialogue you and I might have if you were visiting my salon for the first time. I like to take time to get a full sense of who you are as a new client. Of course, I can form an opinion from looking at you: the way you dress, the manner in which you carry yourself, your accessories, etc. I can observe the color, texture, and density of your hair, see its condition, and judge your current hairstyle.

I have learned that what I can see will only teach me a small sliver of the information I need to know in order to give you your best haircut, your best hair color, and your best overall look. Over the years, I have developed a detailed consultation—actually more of a dialogue—with clients that gives me a fuller picture of who they are.

The dialogue doesn't end with our first time together. It builds from appointment to appointment, month after month, and year after year. Over time, I can track the evolution of a client's life, marked by events large and small. Our dialogue might meander among a wide range of topics, some seemingly unrelated to the theme of hair service, but all helpful clues into getting a clear image of who they are at the time of the service.

Through this dialogue, beginning with our first appointment, I would identify your two most dominant elements from the five elements in Feng Shui. While it will be covered in greater detail later in the book, let me point out that each of us possesses all five elements in our personalities and lifestyles. In Feng Shui, this is called the "basket of elements." Nevertheless, at any point in time two elements will be more dominant: a primary and secondary element. In Feng Shui, these two elements are known as fluctuating elements. The significance of any one element may shift from time to time depending upon any of a number of factors. The maturing process plays a key role in this process; our focus in our twenties is rarely our focus in our fifties. As we travel through the various stages in our lives, from our schooling to our career through our relationships, through the stages of parenting and so on, subtle and stark shifts occur in our focus and our priorities. For example, my priorities from how I dress to how I spend my money and my time are dramatically different today as the father of two small children than they were twenty years ago when I was just starting my career.

These experiences as well as the stages of our life affect the dominant elements in our lives. Whether we have lost our job or gained a new job, lost a loved one through death or divorce or gained a loved one through marriage or the birth of a baby, had our children leave home or had older children return home, these experiences have changed the way we see ourselves. I see it daily in my experience behind the chair in my salons. Whatever affects who we are also affects the way we perceive ourselves and is important in our self-image. The shifts in our life created by outside forces are always accompanied by a shift in our elements. That is why you should revisit this chapter every time a shift has occurred in your life.

Depending on your stage of life, either your personality or your lifestyle will be the more dominant factor. We define personality in terms of who you are on the inside. It is important to consider that while the personality element is a constant, it may sometimes be suppressed because of what you do or what others expect of you. For example, the personality element may become "hidden" at various times in your life, such as when you have dependent children or others living at home.

Our consideration of lifestyle includes hobbies, career, and exercise patterns. Your mate, job, or outside factors influences these traits. These are often fluid traits, changing from time to time.

Your personality and lifestyle may be two different areas in which your elements are expressed, or they may blend seamlessly. Your lifestyle may require you to suppress certain aspects of your personality. Conversely, your personality may lead you to your lifestyle.

For our purposes, we are going to focus on discovering your elements at this point in your life. If you were in my salon, I would have you settle in my chair, sip a cup of green tea, and we would begin our exchange. Now, take a moment to get comfortable, free yourself of distractions, pour yourself a nice cup of green tea, and prepare yourself for this process.

Two of the most important things that I can emphasize about going through this exercise are (1) don't overthink your answers, and (2) be as honest as possible. After all, you are the only one who will see your answers. Bear in mind that there are no right or wrong answers. By being as true to yourself as possible with your answers, you will be able to get the best read as to those qualities that we will be referencing time and time again throughout the rest of the book. Select the answers that best represent your current position. Don't try to work with who you used to be, or what you are striving for, but where you really are today.

So, get a clean sheet of paper and, down the left margin of the paper, write the numbers 1 through 17. Write your answers to the following questions next to the appropriate question numbers on your now numbered sheet. Take a deep, cleansing breath, and let us start.

(Note: For questions 1 and 2, I am not talking about your favorite color, the color of your home, the color you wear the most, your hair color, or even the color of your car. I want to know which color describes you without deliberating or contemplating. If you have difficulty with deciding, think of which color you would want others to use to describe you.)

1. **What color best describes your lifestyle?**
   A. Dark purple to bright pink to red
   B. Brown to orange to yellow
   C. Gray to silver to white and any pastel color
   D. Black to navy to dark blue
   E. All greens, turquoise, and blues except dark blue

2. **What color best describes your personality?**
   A. Dark purple to bright pink to red
   B. Brown to orange to yellow
   C. Gray to silver to white and any pastel color
   D. Black to navy to dark blue
   E. All greens, turquoise, and blues except dark blue

3. **My attitude towards clothing fashion is:**
   A. I love to try the latest trends, the bolder the better.
   B. Comfort is more important to me than trends are.
   C. I have a firm standard for classic styles and rarely deviate from these guidelines.
   D. I tend to prefer chic fashions.
   E. My tastes leans toward unrestricted clothing and sporty styles.

4. **At a party, I tend to:**
   A. Come into my element as the life of the party; more often than not, I am the center of attention.
   B. Settle into intimate conversations with one or two of the other guests with whom I am most comfortable.
   C. Limit my interaction to one or two familiar guests, listening more than speaking.
   D. Prefer to observe the festivities without interaction unless it is discussing the latest book, newest designer, or architect.
   E. Have a nose for a good debate and enjoy lively conversation with a group of people.

5. **I make decisions:**
   A. Quickly, decisively, with no looking back.
   B. Cautiously, but I am committed to them once made.
   C. With little emotion and after an objective weighing of relevant facts.
   D. Reluctantly, sometimes by default, hoping for an intuitive answer.
   E. Efficiently, with an instinctive grasp of the pros and cons.

6. In cooking, my approach is best described as:
A. An adventure; recipes only slow me down.
B. A joyous ritual; I relish the challenge of new dishes and take pleasure in the process of cooking.
C. A process necessary for the end result. I always measure and follow the recipes.
D. Willing to try new gourmet recipes, but just as willing to eat out.
E. Homemade rather than prepared, but it is the company that makes the dinner.

7. I would like for others to see me as:
A. Funny, dramatic, and upbeat.
B. Diplomatic, caring, and agreeable.
C. Organized, disciplined, and responsible.
D. Patient, thoughtful, and sensual.
E. Strong, confident, and successful.

8. My favorite characteristics are my:
A. Creativity and sense of humor.
B. Loyalty and compassion.
C. Efficiency and virtues.
D. Honesty and commitment.
E. Leadership and assertiveness.

9. When I become sick, I tend to:
A. View it as a challenge to overcome.
B. Cocoon until I recuperate.
C. Rely upon my inner strength and focus on healing myself through tried-and-true methods.
D. Look at alternative methods or find a self-help book.
E. Seek advice from my medical providers and adhere to their counsel.

10. The careers that most appeal to me are:
A. Visual arts, performing arts, or teaching.
B. Health care, service, or charity work.
C. Law, engineering, or accounting.
D. Research, psychology, or writing.
E. Management, design, or sales.

11. I respond to change this way:

A. I seek it, as it excites me.

B. I like things the way they are.

C. I want to know why the change is being made and how it will benefit me.

D. I accept the change willingly.

E. I see change as a way to grow.

12. As to my goals, I tend to:

A. Tackle them aggressively at first.

B. Focus on them after I have assisted others in achieving theirs.

C. Methodically identify them, detail the steps, and strategize as to how to reach them.

D. Experience anxiety, achieve them, and go on to something else.

E. Embrace them, but become easily distracted.

13. My temperament is:

A. Mercurial

B. Serene

C. Somewhat aloof

D. Somewhat emotional

E. Assertive

14. In my family, my role is that of:

A. Entertainer

B. Peace keeper

C. Drill sergeant

D. Visionary

E. Motivator

15. My current field of employment is most closely related to:

A. Art/Entertainment/Cooking

B. Health Care/Service/Agriculture

C. Accounting/Law/Engineering

D. Writing/Researching/Consulting

E. Design/Marketing/Sales

16. When I have free time, I most enjoy:
A. Going to a concert, listening to music, or painting.
B. Working around the house, cooking, or visiting friends.
C. Organizing my closets, going to museums, or listening to a lecture.
D. Reading a book, shopping, or reading magazines.
E. Outdoor competitive activities, socializing with groups, or eating out with others.

17. The type of books I most enjoy are:
A. Romance, poetry, or stories of exotic places.
B. Gardening, crafts, or family.
C. Historical, the classics, or serious biographies.
D. Self-help, biographies of artists or creative people, or political commentary.
E. Autobiographies, travel, or adventure.

Go through and count how many times you answered with each letter. The highest number will be your predominant element and the next one will be your secondary element. If you answered every question with the same letter, your predominant and your secondary element are the same. The letters relate to the elements as follows:

A	Fire
B	Earth
C	Metal
D	Water
E	Wood

For example, if you have ten for A, six for D, and one for E, your elements will be Fire/Water.

Now that you know what your dominant elements are, you'll find references to them throughout the rest of this book. If you find that your elements appear to be grossly at odds, either with each other, or with how you're feeling about yourself or the way you are presenting yourself to the world, this book will give you the tools to reconcile the two. As you read the sections that apply to your elements, you will find new insights into how to best express these elements in your hair, makeup, and fashion.

While some may dismiss this test as too simplistic to determine a person's element, I have tested these questions on thousands of my clients for the last ten years and have had amazing results. I have had clients cry in my chair as I was sharing insights about them, based upon my questioning and an application of the principles behind the elements. My clients have stated that I nailed their personality and lifestyle traits correctly. The results have been virtually one hundred percent accurate. It has made a difference in my relationships with my clients and in the life of my clients. If you take the time to study your answers and learn about your element, it will make a difference in your life also.

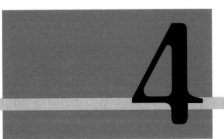

4 The Bagua

The Bagua is derived from the *I Ching*, or Chinese Book of Changes. The Bagua describes the eight basic building blocks of the *I Ching*, called *trigrams*. Each trigram is associated with specific "treasures" in life, such as health, wealth, and love. In the practice of Feng Shui, the Bagua is used to map out homes, rooms, and office buildings. It is also used to locate the areas that correspond to the various treasures, giving every part of the building significance and meaning. According to Feng Shui, the good fortune of the inhabitants is significantly strengthened when the Bagua of their home or workplace has been properly mapped out and enhanced. I have found that when my clients are aware of the eight trigrams that affect their lives, they have more power to change any area that is not in balance.

The discipline of Feng Shui is about honoring you as a temple and looking at the complete person as a temple. I can assist you to make changes on the outside to reflect how you perceive yourself on the inside. You, however, are the only one who can make any changes in your life's direction. Just as treatments or exercise systems provide excellent results if followed regularly, the Bagua can also assist in providing positive results in your life. The Bagua checklists in this chapter are for you to use to analyze your life and influences.

Throughout my consultations with my clients, I ask various questions related to these areas of influence. From my clients' responses, I learn details about my clients' areas of influence and the value that is placed on them. I ask that you find a quiet space and spend time reflecting on the questions in this chapter. This Bagua will only be useful if you examine your life and make any changes that you decide are necessary.

The successful results produced by the Bagua occur from combining two forces. The first is the timeless wisdom that the *I Ching* provides. The second is the user's serious intention to produce a positive change in her life. According to the Chinese, the physical world is a map for our emotional life and what is observed in each area can express much about a person's internal life. The Bagua is an ancient tool that can be used to help determine what specific areas in life are in harmony, what areas need to be enhanced, and which areas need to be balanced.

Bagua

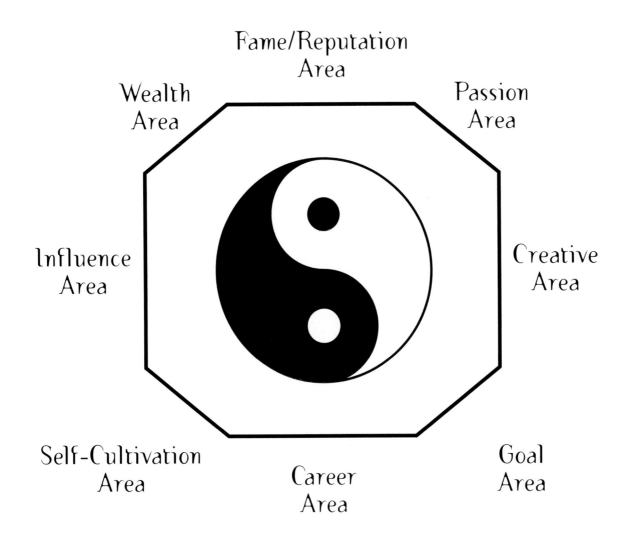

Fame/Reputation
Area

Wealth
Area

Passion
Area

Influence
Area

Creative
Area

Self-Cultivation
Area

Career
Area

Goal
Area

Fame or Reputation

The first influence is your Fame or Reputation Area. Fame has different meanings according to the individual and culture. The dictionary defines fame as "widespread and illustrious reputation; renown or your public reputation or estimation." We hear about fleeting fame and the price of fame. Paraphrasing Andy Warhol's often-quoted notion, everyone will have fifteen minutes of fame. Some confuse fame with narcissism, which means you have achieved fame only in your own mind. We all have fame or a reputation that precedes us. In this aspect of the Bagua, I use Fame to mean what you have accomplished and/or want to accomplish. For this exercise, it is also important to think about your values.

1. What are you known for?
2. What do you want to be known for?
3. How important is honesty and integrity in your life? Explain.
4. How do you want to be described or remembered by the following people?
   • Friends
   • Mother/Father
   • Significant Other
   • Coworkers
   • Children
   • Siblings
5. How do you visualize yourself?
6. What contributions have you made that set you apart?
7. What awards or recognition have you received? For what?
8. What are your values?
9. Where would you like to make changes in your life?
10. What are the steps you will utilize to achieve these changes?

"Some people fear gaining fame
the way pigs fear gaining weight."

—*Chinese Proverb*

Passion

The second influence is your Passion Area. Passion is defined as any intense, extreme, or overpowering emotion or feeling. It is easy to see the difference between people who have passion for what they do and those who merely go to work. I believe that when you have passion for what you do, you never go to work. When an artist has passion, the creation has energy. Think about the difference in listening to a speaker who is passionate about his topic as opposed to a speaker who is merely mouthing information. Look at the difference in someone cooking with passion and love instead of just cooking food to satisfy hunger pains. Passion is the zest or the energy that people pour into their beliefs, values, and art. The passion that you express about a project or endeavor is very contagious to those around you. Someone who is passionate about life remains youthful through all experiences.

1. What are your interests?
2. How passionate are you about your choice of a career?
3. How do you show your passion to others?
4. What really excites you?
5. How much of the day are you passionate about life?
6. Describe your passion level in the following areas:
   - Family
   - Knowledge
   - Visual Arts
   - Performing Arts
   - Politics
   - Spirituality
   - Sports
   - Relationships
7. What can you do to express more passion in life?

"Nothing great has been and nothing great can be accomplished without Passion."

—G. Wilhelm Fredrich Hegel

"Creative work is play..."

—*Stephen Nachmanovitch*

Creativity

The third influence is the Creative Area. Creativity means unlimited possibilities or thinking outside of the box and is characterized by originality of thought and execution. I believe that daydreaming is a requirement for releasing your creative energy. For some of us, we lost the luxury of daydreaming when we were young as we were taught to focus in our classes and where being creative was limited to art classes.

Creativity requires you to stay young at heart and be willing to take a risk. Without failure, there would be no standard for success. In my profession, creativity is the driving force in creating cuts and colors for my clients. I can teach new designers cutting and coloring techniques—the technical aspect. The techniques may be perfect but without creativity and passion, it is just a haircut. I believe we never lose our ability to be creative, but sometimes we don't honor it or practice it. We need to be free to create. This influence is extremely important for having good Chi or energy.

1. What does being creative mean to you?
2. How creative are you in the following areas:
   - Cooking
   - Decorating
   - Clothing
   - Accessories
   - Speech
   - Hobbies
   - Social life
   - Entertaining
   - Career
   - Relationships
   - Hair/Makeup
3. What are you doing daily as a creative outlet?
4. Describe your most creative experience.
5. How creative is your life?

Goals

The fourth influence is the Goal Area. Goals are defined as something toward which effort or movement is directed; an end or objective. Goals serve as a map to keep us on track, to remind us of where we are going and why. For unorganized people, goals edge us toward more planning for success. They bring discipline into our lives. They also serve as milestones of our lives and remind us of our achievements. It helps to record your goals in a journal or to write them where you will see them daily or weekly. In our chaotic world, we often become too busy completing the task of working and caring for our families that we fail to think about our goals. I have found that going over my goals the first thing in the morning or the last thing at night keeps them fresh in my mind. Often, we make unrealistic or unachievable goals so we have excuses as to why we didn't reach them. This exercise is to assist you in staying on track for achieving your goals for yourself. When pondering your goals for this exercise, you should consider your goals in terms of daily goals, one year goals, and three year goals or for the timeline most meaningful to you.

1. What are your personal goals?
2. What are your professional goals?
3. Have you achieved any of your goals? If so, which?
4. What goal would you like to achieve first or next?
5. Do you have goals concerning the following? If so, what are those goals,
   and what are your plans and timeline for achieving them?
   • Your overall look
   • Your hair
   • Your skin
   • Exercise
   • Your weight
   • Your nails
   • Your health
6. What are your goals in regards to your relationships?
7. Which of your goals will require more than one year to achieve?
8. What is your routine for visiting your goals? Do you have them written down
   and/or a check list to document the attainment of a milestone?

"The tragedy of life doesn't lie in not reaching our goal.
The tragedy lies in having no goal to reach."

—Benjamin E. Mays

Career

The fifth influence is the Career Area. Career is defined as "the course or progress of events, especially in a person's life and one's lifework; profession." Often, we associate having a career with receiving a regular paycheck with a title and career path. However, I want to broaden that definition. If you are an artist but don't sell your work, or if you are a stay-at-home parent, that is still your career. You have selected to make your art or your home and your children your career. We ultimately define what a career is to us and how much of our time we are willing to expend to achieve our goals whether they be financial or some other measure.

1. How do you define your career? Or does it define you?
2. How much does your career affect your lifestyle?
3. Where are you in your career?
   - Are you just starting?
   - What is your position in your career?
4. What education or training was required for your career choice?
5. Will you make any changes in your career? If so, what and why?
6. How does your career affect the way you dress? Your hair, makeup, etc.?
7. How involved are you with your community?
8. Do you serve as a mentor for anyone? How? Who was your mentor?
9. How many hours a day are you involved with your career?

"Work to me is a sacred thing."

—Margaret Bourke-White

Self-Cultivation

The sixth influence is the Self-Cultivation Area. We're living in an era of self-cultivation and self-improvement. Self-help sections in bookstores have drastically expanded and the growth in gyms and personal trainers has exploded throughout the country. Everything seems to focus on improving Me and about Me. One would think this influence would have created a generation of happy and fulfilled individuals; however, it seems the opposite has occurred. Individuals compare themselves with others and never seem happy with who they are or sometimes don't even know who they are. My interpretation on this influence has a different twist: it is not only to make you reach your full potential, it is also to make you happier and enjoy life. I urge you to live in the Now and to bring balance into your life. To learn how to reduce or live with stress in your life requires you to focus on the routines in your daily life. This is the importance of the Self-Cultivation Area.

1. How much time do you focus on exercise?
2. How involved are you in your nutrition?
3. Do you eat only because you are hungry? Are you aware of what you are eating?
4. How concerned are you about organic foods and health supplements?
5. Do you have medical checkups regularly?
6. How much time do you allocate for enjoying nature and the beauty that surrounds you?
7. How much time do you spend meditating, praying, or exploring who you are and your relationship with nature?
8. What was the last book you read or listened to on tape?
9. Did you read it for information, work, or pleasure?
10. How often do you attend an event of the arts: theatre, movies, concerts, art galleries, or museums?
11. Where was the last place you traveled to for pleasure or work?
12. What did you see that inspired you?
13. If you could be anywhere in the world, where would you be and why?
14. How much time do you spend dreaming?
15. How are you a happier person now than last year? Why? If not, why not?

"Men who work cannot dream, and wisdom comes to us in dreams."

—Smohalla, Nez Prezi Tribal Leader

> "It would be difficult to exaggerate the degree to which we are influenced by those we influence."
>
> —*Eric Hoffer*

Influence

The seventh influence is the Influence Area. We cannot escape the influences that play an important role in our lives. Even a hermit's choice of shelter, clothing, and food are influenced by the environment! We all have influences whether we acknowledge them or not; advertising, television, media, music, society, work, family, religion, and mentors are all possible areas of influence. It is important to recognize these influences and to realize that we have the power to control the extent of their effects.

1. Age is a major influence for many people. How much does your age influence your decisions? Why?
2. Describe the way you see yourself. Are you brilliant, witty, charming, shy, aloof, happy-go-lucky, fat, thin, tall, short, old, young? Remember that others usually see you as you see yourself. You project that image. Write a short description of you.
3. How do your children influence what you wear in clothing and your hairstyle?
4. How much does your significant other influence your clothing or hairstyle?
5. When you look in the mirror, what is your best feature?
6. What would you like to change about yourself? Why?
7. How do your friends influence you?
8. When you walk into a room, what energy do you carry with you?
9. How are you influenced by where you live and what you do?
10. Who do you influence and how?

Wealth

The eighth influence is the Wealth Area. Wealth has been defined as "great abundance of valuable possessions; riches or a great amount; a wealth of learning." I believe that every person defines her own wealth. The *I Ching* states that life is ever-changing and never-changing. A person's definition of wealth also changes according to experiences and the stages in life. Wealth does play an important role in our actions and our self image. Our focus on achieving wealth limits or expands our horizons and opportunities. It is important that you think about your definition of wealth and the amount of time you are willing to spend in acquiring it.

1. How do you identify wealth?
2. How often do you travel or vacation? Is this important to you?
3. What is success to you?
4. What defines wealth for you? Money, homes, jewelry, children, family, good health, love, a great job, knowledge, education, freedom to enjoy life, friendships, luxury cars, yachts, town homes, travel? You know what makes you feel successful.
5. Have you invested in something that can be lost or something that is long lasting?
6. How important is happiness to your definition of wealth?
7. What role does being happy play in your life?
8. Has your idea about wealth changed in the last five years? If so, how?
9. Do you have a plan for achieving your definition of wealth? If so, what is it?

"People are tested by wealth,
just as gold is tested by fire."

—*Chinese Proverb*

Yin/Yang Balance

The center of the Bagua is the Yin/Yang symbol in which is everything in balance. No one can answer these questions for you. If you are truly interested in making your life better and in being in control of your life, you have a choice. Nothing will change your life but your choices, which begin with your intention. The information contained in this chapter was created as a tool to assist you in understanding yourself. This is a step toward identifying yourself through the five elements.

5 Yin/Yang Energy

To be able to understand the nature of your own energy, you must understand the power of Yin and Yang (pronounced "yen" and "yon") as well as the importance of the five elements.

In China, the theory of the five elements coexisted early with the theory of the two forces of Yin and Yang. In Chinese philosophy, balance and harmony manifest when the two polar energy forces of Yin and Yang exist simultaneously within everything in the universe. The first lesson about Yin and Yang is in understanding their cyclical character. They transform into one another. At the extreme of Yin, the seed of Yang is born.

The second lesson in understanding Yin and Yang is that there is a negative-to-positive polarity. Yin and Yang must be interpreted as a highly dynamic process where the two areas are constantly changing and keeping the whole in balance. They dance between each other. One does not exist without the other. In Feng Shui, you are meant to have both Yin and Yang energies, as they complement one another to achieve harmony.

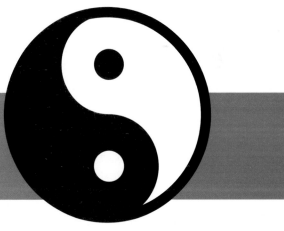

Yin/Yang

Yin is female and Yang is male. Neither moves nor acts without consequences to the other. The line that separates the sides is fluid and moves depending on the balance between the two. In each half is the presence of its opposite to remind us that in every element of maleness, there exists a bit of the female and vice versa.

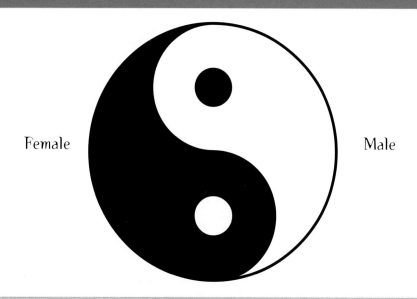

Female   Male

Yin
Female

Yang
Male

Yin (Female)	Yang (Male)
Soft	Angular
Reserved	Outgoing
Sour	Sweet
Sad	Happy
Moon	Sun
Quiet	Loud
Passive	Aggressive
Cool	Warm
Dark	Light
Curved	Straight
Earth	Sky
Inward	Outward
Low	High

In order to illustrate the Yin/Yang principle in the real world, a few examples may be useful. Each of these illustrates an extreme:

A female professional model whose life and livelihood depend on her beauty and femininity would be an extreme of Yin. Should there be a threat to her status or beauty (such as through aging) her response might be much more Yang (aggressive) than that of a woman whose focus wasn't so Yin.

A male body builder with tremendous strength and body mass (Yang) would experience a greater blow to his strength were he to come down with an illness than someone who exercises more moderately. The bodybuilder will become relatively weaker (Yin) and may find recovery more difficult.

To understand the importance of the five elements within Yin and Yang, we must look at the extreme and moderate characteristics within each element. Most people aren't comfortable admitting or acknowledging the most severe or unflattering characteristics of themselves, but you can take comfort in knowing also that we each possess traits across the board. This occurs not only in our most dominant element, but within the basket of five elements as well. The task, therefore, is to take a realistic assessment of which characteristics most accurately describe who you are today.

When a client comes to my salon, I do this assessment visually. I look at the way she walks and carries herself, the spirit that she expresses, her handshake (is it confident or tentative?), and the way she looks at me (does she meet my eyes?).

In defining the basic characteristics for self-assessment in this chapter, I found it much easier to reduce it to a few descriptions. Please note that in the chapters on each of the five elements, I describe the personality of each element with more depth.

In Chapter 3: It's All About You, you determined your dominant element. Use the Element Barometers to determine whether your dominant element is or is not in balance.

Look at your dominant element. Check which column best describes yourself in your life right now. This is not what you want to be, it's who you really are, right now. Being honest with yourself about this will help you determine whether your element needs to be enhanced (strengthened), harmonized (suppressed or calmed), or balanced (stabilized), and you can use the luo pans at the end of the chapter to help you figure out how to do that.

The column numbered 2 is Yin Extreme and needs to be harmonized with a productive element (the element that in traditional Feng Shui "produces," as Wood produces Fire, Fire produces Earth, Earth produces Metal, and so on). The column numbered 4 is Yin Moderate and needs to be enhanced by adding the same element. The column numbered 6 is Yang Moderate and needs to be harmonized with a calming element. The column numbered 8 is Yang Extreme and needs to be balanced with its opposite element.

Fire

2 Yin Extreme
- I look for excitement
- I have trouble making up my mind—I don't want to close off any choices
- I'm feeling socially burned out lately

Harmonize with Wood

4 Yin Moderate
- I'm flexible, easily able to change course
- I feel enthusiastic and positive
- When I'm around others, I feel energized and charismatic

Enhance with Fire

6 Yang Moderate
- I'm passionate about life
- I'm excitable, full of enthusiasm, quick to respond
- I'm not always aware of others' needs

Harmonize with Earth

8 Yang Extreme
- I can be hot tempered and dramatic
- I'm eager to fight for what I believe in
- I find myself burning the candle at both ends

Balance with Water

Earth

2 Yin Extreme
- I need attachment to other people or to my possessions
- I like to feel safe
- I have a hard time saying "no"

Harmonize with Fire

4 Yin Moderate
- I am a creature of habit
- I'm realistic about my life
- I'm persistent and willing to work hard

Enhance with Earth

6 Yang Moderate
- I am steadfast and loyal
- I like to be consistent and do the same things the same way
- I am polite and have very good manners

Harmonize with Metal

8 Yang Extreme
- I sometimes dig in my heels
- I don't like change unless it's my idea
- I'd rather keep things the way they are

Balance with Wood

Metal

2 Yin Extreme
- I don't feel much like socializing lately
- I am cautious and careful in making decisions
- I am oblivious to those around me

Harmonize with Earth

4 Yin Moderate
- I like to have everything around me very organized
- I want to weigh all my options before making any changes
- I'm thorough and dependable

Enhance with Metal

6 Yang Moderate
- I am efficient and expedient
- I make quick decisions
- I'm very focused

Harmonize with Water

8 Yang Extreme
- I am a perfectionist and can be picky
- Once I've made up my mind, I stick to my guns
- I don't tune in to my emotional side much

Balance with Fire

Water

2 Yin Extreme
- I feel better if I get a lot of reassurance
- I'm very sympathetic to others and sometimes they take advantage of me
- My feelings get hurt pretty easily and I lack clear boundaries

Harmonize with Metal

4 Yin Moderate
- I like other people to help me make decisions
- My emotions are pretty close to the surface
- I'm reflective and insightful

Enhance with Water

6 Yang Moderate
- It's easy for me to go with the flow
- I'm agreeable and easy to be around
- I'm good at seeing all sides of a conflict and helping people get through it

Harmonize with Wood

8 Yang Extreme
- I'm private and keep secrets well
- I can be too critical of myself and others sometimes
- I can be temperamental

Balance with Earth

Wood

2 Yin Extreme
- I feel scattered lately
- I'm usually the one to end a relationship
- If things aren't going my way, I'd just as soon move on

Harmonize with Water

4 Yin Moderate
- I absorb new information quickly and easily
- I'm gentle and accepting with others
- I'm good at handling pressure, I'm a good leader

Enhance with Wood

6 Yang Moderate
- I am optimistic but I don't like to be alone
- I can be impatient with others
- I'm athletic but not artistic

Harmonize with Fire

8 Yang Extreme
- I'm sometimes hasty or quick to judge
- In relationships I'm usually the one to make the first move
- I can be demanding and sometimes hard to please

Balance with Metal

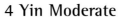

Yin/Yang Energy

The Luo Pan

The luo pan is used as a guide to assist you in determining the proper techniques to enhance, harmonize, or balance your elements once you have identified them and determined whether they are in or out of balance.

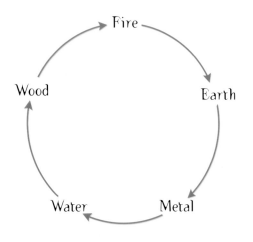

Harmonize
Productive Luo Pan
Yin Extreme 2: Your element needs to be strengthened gradually. You will add the productive element.

Harmonize

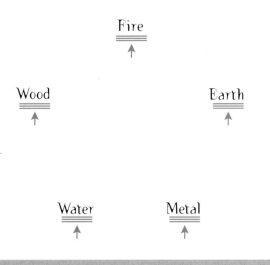

Enhance
Enhance Luo Pan
Yin Moderate 4: You want to give expression to an understated element by spotlighting it.

Enhance

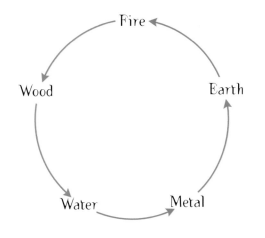

Exhaustive

Exhaustive Luo Pan
Yang Moderate 6: Your element needs to be weakened or diminished slightly. You will use the exhaustive element.

Exhaustive

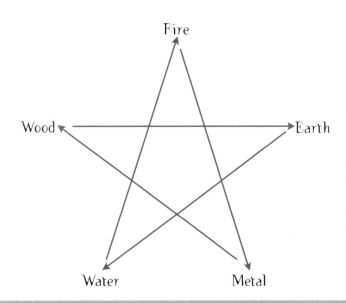

Balance

Balance Luo Pan
Yang Extreme 8: You need to stabilize your element by adding the opposite element.

Balance

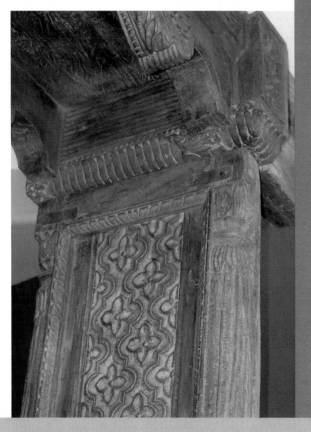

6 Fire Element

A Fire person is charismatic and has extraordinary energy. Fire types are usually at the heart of the action; others are drawn to their engaging personality. Fire types react without thinking and change their minds just as quickly. If the fire is not contained, fire energy changes into a flash fire and is depleted while being destructive. Fire personality traits can become out of control when surrounded by other Fire types and Fire surroundings.

With Fire types, there is no in-between; something is either fabulous or horrible. A new style, new fad, new music group, new restaurant—new, new, new—Fire types experience it first. A Fire type would not excel in the military or under stringent regulations, as restraints and rules are unacceptable. If a Fire person were forced into this kind of environment, she would become despondent. Lots of clear space gives Fire room to express and create. A small room or space with clutter or lots of knickknacks tends to make Fire feel irritable and smothered. Someone who is constantly pushing the rules and going out on the edge with any endeavor usually has Fire traits.

Surrounded by bright color and unusual objects, Fire types have interesting, fun homes or rooms. They love being the center of attention whether at work, at home, or with friends. They are great at brainstorming and extremely creative—especially when there are no rules. Fire types bring creativity to the business world and are great leaders or business owners when they are in balance.

Fire types like to attract attention with their dress, hair, accessories, or talent. When they are good, they are very good. They are very passionate at whatever they choose to experience. As designers, they push the envelope and think outside the box. It is this same enthusiasm that helps to catapult the Fire type to the top of the heap as an athlete, artist, singer, or actor. Fire movie or television producers are legendary for their antics on the set. They like to be in charge and will go to any extent to get the end result, which will be fantastic.

A Fire type is an excellent person to ask for advice about the best restaurant, play, "in spot," or movie. Fire personalities are usually very bright, but do not respond to conventional measures of intelligence. In school, grades may not be a reflection of their knowledge. Fire types respond quickly—and think about it later. They are the types to be around when you need immediate feedback.

The Fire type takes this same enthusiasm and excitement into her lifestyle and career. There is no certain occupation that a Fire type might select; however, it is highly unlikely a Fire type would select a position that would involve total focus on details and organization such as an accountant or bookkeeper. A desk or work area that is filled with stacks of work-in-progress mixed with ideas on small notes would usually belong to a Fire type. Fire types can multitask easily, but they run the risk of not completing any of the tasks on time. It is the passion that one would take to the position or hobby that would define the Fire type. A Fire artist creates with bold splashes of color that attracts and excites the senses. A teacher is usually thought of as being an Earth element because nurturing and caring traits are needed. How fortunate for those of us who were lucky enough to have had a Fire professor to share his/her passion and spark our interest.

Within each element, Yin and Yang energies exist. On the Element Barometer in Chapter 5: Ying/Yang Energy, I have listed characteristics that will assist you in knowing whether you need to enhance, harmonize, or balance the element. If the Fire element is hidden or Yin Extreme 2, you need to add the Wood element to encourage more expression. When the Yin is Moderate 4, you need to enhance the Fire. If the Yang is Moderate 6, you need to calm the Fire, not suppress it, and I recommend adding some Earth element into your life. When the Fire element is too extreme, Yang 8, I recommend using the Water element to balance or control the Fire. The degree of Fire element that we express can be compared to the different types of Fires in our lives. A wildfire is unpredictable and extremely hard to contain. That would be similar to a Yang Fire 8 on the Element Barometer. A Yang Fire 6 would be similar to a fire somewhat contained in a fireplace. A Yin Fire 4 would be much like the fire on a cooking stove that is controlled and responds to the knobs that control it. To increase the fire, you would turn up the knob and add more fire. A Yin Fire 2 would be similar to a dying fire. It is still a fire although very faint. Add Wood to feed the fire and give it life.

Using Feng Shui principles designed to bring balance or create a flow of good Chi, I take into consideration not only your haircut, hair color, makeup, body type, and face shape, but also your hobbies, your lifestyle, your exercise patterns, meditation, clothing, and accessories. All of these things affect you and the image you portray.

When I prescribe the look that will best reflect how you perceive yourself, I also make recommendations for other factors that influence your life. Some of the recommendations or changes will be evident almost immediately such as haircut, hair color, and makeup. The other changes will involve more participation and will evolve as you are the one in charge of implementing that part of your life. The amount of change will depend upon your dedication.

Makeup for the Fire Element

You can certainly use more expressive, bold colors as well as techniques. The only restriction is your skin tone. Makeup is a way to create a new look that can change with your moods. I recommend selecting strong true colors for eyes and lips. Your element is one of the few that can make a strong statement with bold colors.

Porcelain Skin Tone

Emphasize the eyes with a gray or blue eyeliner, blue and purple eye shadows. Your lips could be deeper shades of purple or sparkling pinks.

Milky Skin Tone

Think shiny with golds, rich auburn, and shades of browns and greens on eyes. Lips should be moist with nudes and peach colors.

Honey Skin Tone

Use strong shades of oranges, cinnamon or complementary strong pinks on eyes and lips. Use a shimmer across the cheekbones.

Olive Skin Tone

Go for strong smoky eyes with deeper true colors used such as gray or black. Paint the lips strong with berry colors.

Ebony Skin Tone

Boldly use strong colors for the eyes. Berry, deep red, or orange can be used on the lips.

Ruby Skin Tones

Sultry eyes with brown, gold, or rust along with the same colors on lips.

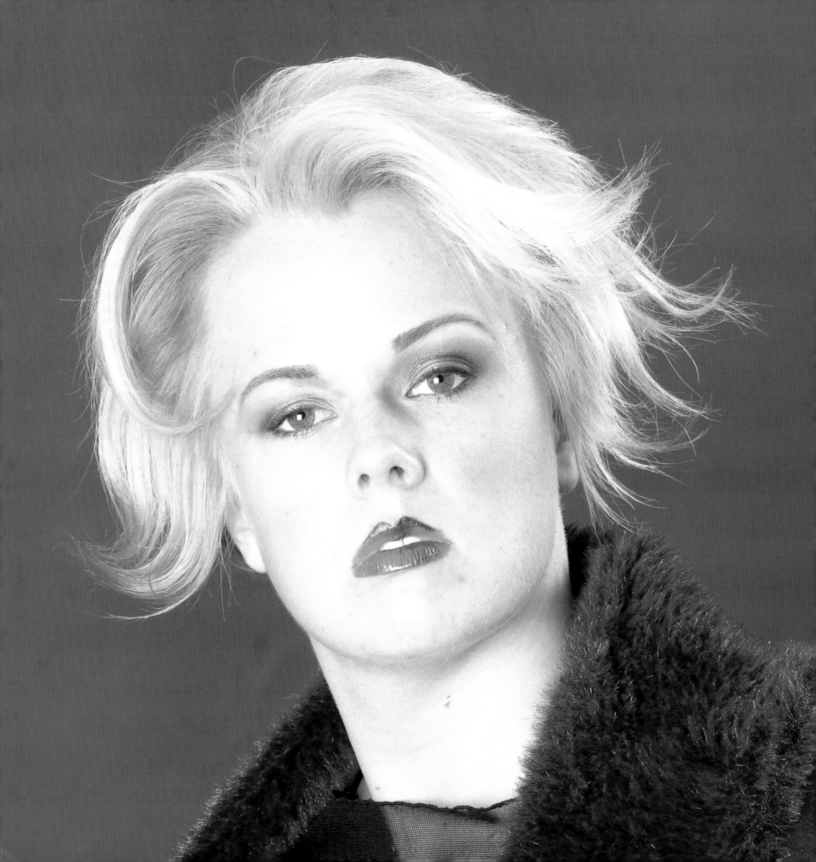

Fire/Fire

If you selected Fire for your personality and Fire for your lifestyle, then your elements are listed as Fire/Fire. The unstoppable double Fire! The intensity of Fire/Fire people usually extends to all that they do. Whether it's storming through new information or sampling a new experience, the double Fire tends to race through life like a wildfire through straw. When given a new project or task, they leap at the opportunity to forge ahead and explore new territory. Fire/Fire types are not the easiest people to be around; however, they are some of the most exciting. Fire/Fire types will never be labeled as an enabler because they become impatient with anyone demanding too much of their time and energy. Fire/Fire types will stimulate you and invigorate you but only on their terms.

Harmonize Fire/Fire 2

If you measured Yin Extreme or 2 on the Element Barometer, this indicates that even though you are a double Fire you may not be honoring the flame that burns inside. You may be trying to be whatever is "acceptable." You need to add Wood to feed the Fire and make it more expressive. The Wood element type is more outgoing, social, and loves to be outdoors or on the go. Often a Fire type will remain aloof or would rather be alone if there is no outlet for creativity or passion. By adding Wood to feed the Fire, you increase the expression of what's inside. Think about how you spend your leisure time. I recommend seeking a release of your creative talents through the arts, hobbies, or outdoor activities. The goal with Feng Shui is to bring you into balance. Refer to Chapter 12: Skin Tone and Hair Color for specific color formulations that your stylist can use to enhance your Fire element.

Haircut to Harmonize Fire/Fire 2

Harmonize the Fire with Wood by adding random texture to create uneven pieces for a tousled style. Movement is the key for this cut and style. Wood feeds Fire and encourages more creativity. A Wood cut has texture and movement within structure. The style will be more controlled than a Fire cut. A Wood cut for short hair will be more textured at the ends while a Wood cut for longer hair will create more movement by adding rounded layers. Creating a Wood cut for curly hair allows the curls to move and be natural within the cut. Depending on the face shape, hair can be long or short with curls. The key component to the look will be the bounce or movement in the style. Refer to Chapter 11 for the best cut, length, and cutting techniques for you.

Hair color to Harmonize Fire/Fire 2

Make the colors rich and deep. If you are a level five on the color chart, (see Chapter 12: Skin Tone and Hair Color) you can select from levels three through eight according to your skin tone. The highlighting techniques need to show more separation between the weaves for a tousled color. The techniques would be two to four pieces per pickup. Use two to three different colors in highlighting as it will add richness and depth to the color. The placement of the highlights depends on your face shape (see Chapter 11: Hairstyling for Your Body Type, Face Shape, and Facial Features).

Enhance Fire/Fire 4

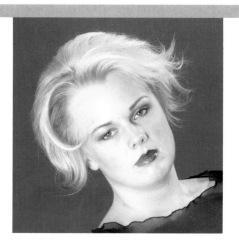

If you measured Yin Moderate or 4 on the Element Barometer, this indicates that you need to enhance your Fire with Fire for more expression. Since you are more comfortable and confident with your creative and passionate traits, you are perfect to have a Fire color/cut and/or makeup. Your career and lifestyle will set the limits. Be bold and express your energetic creativity. Make certain that you include opportunities to honor your adventurous desires.

Haircut to Enhance Fire/Fire 4

Enhance the Fire with an edgy, disconnected, choppy, or over-textured style. Remember the cut and the length will depend on your face shape and facial features. With any cut, texture, or length, I recommend a dramatic style. It may be disconnected or an asymmetric cut. Think of a Picasso painting and you will see the possibilities for a creative cut. If you have curly hair, your cut will depend on the amount of curl and wave. It will be hard to have an edgy cut for extremely curly hair unless you decide to straighten it. Strive for an explosive or bold cut to release the Fire inside.

Hair color to Enhance Fire/Fire 4

Colors can be bold, just make certain that you are using the color chart for your skin tone as well as element. You can be daring and exciting with your color. The highlighting techniques you would choose will be bold. When selecting highlights, you are not striving for subtlety. You can certainly wear the latest fads if your lifestyle permits.

Harmonize Fire/Fire 6

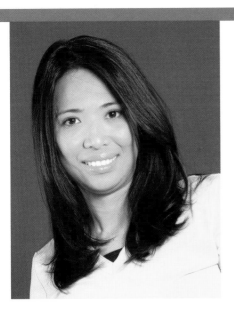

If you measured Yang Moderate or 6 on the Element Barometer, indicating too much Fire in your personality, add Earth to control the Fire. Earth types are calm and enjoy nature. The old saying "Stop and smell the roses" serves as a reminder for the Fire element who usually rushes through the day. Gardening, walking, or any activity that requires you to slow down, will help to balance the Yang Fire type. I recommend introducing the Earth element into either the cut or the color. Earth can stop the Fire or keep it under control depending upon how much is added. We don't want to destroy the Fire, only control it.

Haircut to Harmonize Fire/Fire 6

Harmonize with Earth by cutting uneven pieces throughout the hair for support and texture. The cut should have expression with a natural look. Earth cuts are characteristically very natural and blunt. However, since you only want to ease the Fire, I would make certain the cut has uneven pieces that give it a more exciting look. This look is a mixture of Earth element mixed with the sass of Fire. The length of your haircut depends upon your face shape. See Chapter 11 for the best cut for you. For the Earth element, we are adding interest to the natural cut.

Hair color to Harmonize Fire/Fire 6

Strive for a softer look in highlighting by using Earth techniques. The weaves should be more natural with four to six pieces used for each pickup. The placement depends upon your face shape. See Chapter 12: Skin Tone and Hair Color for coloring techniques. While you want Earth coloring techniques and colors, it is vital that you keep the colors rich and exciting. Too much Earth will dampen the creativity and brilliance of Fire.

Balance Fire/Fire 8

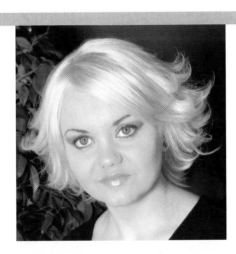

If you measured Yang Extreme or 8 on the Element Barometer, Fire/Fire is totally out of control. I recommend calming the Fire by adding balance with the Water element. Water exhausts Fire or, if added gradually, can calm it. Water types are more reflective and think before acting. Water techniques create a flowing movement that is subtle and sensual. Fire techniques tend to be more choppy, explosive, and sexual. Adding Water still allows creativity to be expressed but in a more sophisticated manner. I recommend more reading and meditating to calm the Yang Extreme 8 Fire. Also, allocating time for your spiritual needs will enrich the life of a Fire/Fire and assist in bringing your Chi into balance.

Fire Element

Haircut to Balance Fire/Fire 8

Balance with Water by making the hair flirty and not over-textured. The haircut needs to have a kick or outward movement for a more fashionable flair. A longer cut would have flowing softer movement with the texture at the ends. With shorter hair, Water cuts tend to be more sleek and chic. The texture adds support for volume or movement. Refer to Chapter 11: Hairstyling for Your Body Type, Face Shape, and Facial Features for best haircut length and styles.

Hair color to Balance Fire/Fire 8

Take the color to a more chic tone by selecting colors from the Water color chart. With Water, you can select colors four levels down from your natural level or five levels up depending on your skin tone. Use Water highlighting techniques by picking up two to seven pieces depending on the texture of your hair. For curly hair, you will want more separated pieces by using two to four per pickup. I like to use two to three colors when highlighting or lowlighting. This adds more excitement to the color.

Fire/Earth

A Fire/Earth combination is independent and enjoys being around others, but doesn't require company to excel. Sometimes a Fire/Earth may stay out of contact with friends for long periods of time; however, when they reconnect they pick up right where they left off. They are great partners as they are creative, exciting, and nurturing. Fire/Earth types burn up a lot of energy as Fire types go into everything with great gusto and Earth types are very caring and give their energy willingly. They tend to be focused and achieve all of their goals. The Fire element wants to be free while the Earth element seeks to be around others upon their own terms. The Fire/Earth types love to travel and see exciting places, but they are willing to wait until they can go first class. Fire/Earth is creative with great ideas and this winning combination has the determination to complete any task they begin.

Fire/Earth types can be every expressive and artistic in any endeavor. As an artist, the expression would not just be in painting, drawing, or sculpture; but it would carry over into cooking, gardening, and sewing. These types do not paint or plant by the numbers, but they are willing to be daring in their gardening and sewing. Their work becomes a canvas for their artistic element. Even though these types may be nurturing and love to cook and care for the family or loved ones, they never just cook a meal. They are the first to try new recipes and substitute exciting ingredients to make fabulous new creations.

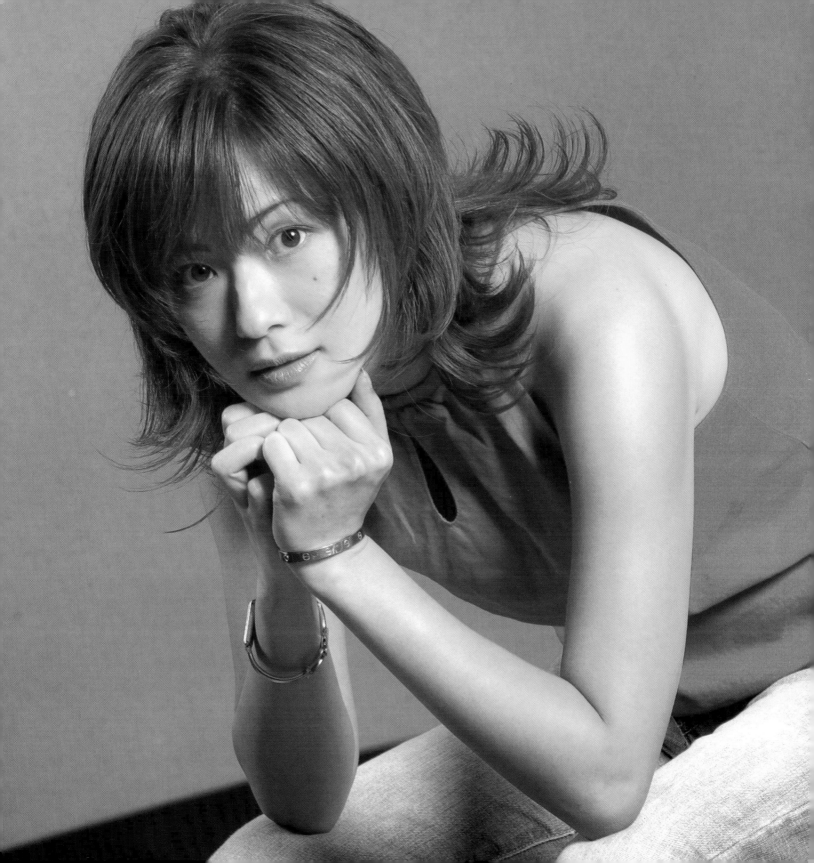

Harmonize Fire/Earth 2

If you measured Yin Extreme or 2 on the Element Barometer, this indicates that your Fire/Earth elements are hidden or not expressed. I recommend harmonizing with the Wood element. Wood will feed the Fire for more expression and still honor the Earth influence. Adding Wood will allow the Fire/Earth to express their artistic talents in a more social setting. Wood types encourage an optimistic outlook on life as they always see their tea cup as half full. This same attitude is seen in the lifestyles and hobbies of the Wood types. Wood types are outgoing and always moving forward.

Haircut to Harmonize Fire/Earth 2

Harmonize with Wood by cutting into the hair for texture. The short hair will support the longer hair much as grass supports. Think of the wind blowing grass and the subtle movements. There is still room for expression in the style, but it is non-threatening to the artistic Fire/Earth type. Refer to Chapter 11: Hairstyling for Your Body Type, Face Shape, and Facial Features for the best length and styles.

Hair color to Harmonize Fire/Earth 2

Harmonize with Wood highlighting techniques. Use two to four pieces for each pickup. Refer to Chapter 11: Hairstyling for Your Body Type, Face Shape, and Facial Features on coloring techniques and application for face shape, and for Wood element tips. I recommend using richer or deeper colors. Check Chapter 12: Skin Tone and Hair Color on hair color according to skin tone.

Enhance Fire/Earth 4

If you measured Yin Moderate or 4 on the Element Barometer, you need to add more Fire techniques and colors to reflect your hidden element. You want to release the Fire while respecting the Earth influence. Your overall look will be more fun and artistic, but not as much as a Fire/Fire. The flair of the Fire will be tempered by the natural style of the Earth element.

Haircut to Enhance Fire/Earth 4

Enhance the Fire side with your hairstyle by having uneven pieces that are disconnected and kicky, not smooth. The Earth influence will set the boundaries as to how artistic and free-flowing your haircut will be. You set the limits as a Fire type has no limits in fashion. If you select a Fire haircut and color or highlights, you would want to use Earth makeup techniques. Refer to Chapter 11:

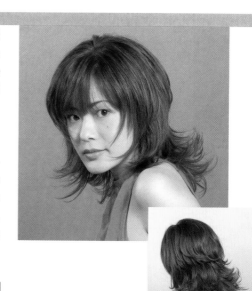

Hairstyling for Your Body Type, Face Shape, and Facial Features for cutting recommendations.

Hair color to Enhance Fire/Earth 4

Brighten the color while still respecting the natural level. With the Fire element, you can wear any level of color depending on your skin tone. If you add slicing singular as well as back to back, you will have bold color. See Chapter 12: Skin Tone and Hair Color as well as Chapter 11: Hairstyling for Your Body Type, Face Shape, and Facial Features for color and highlighting placement.

Harmonize Fire/Earth 6

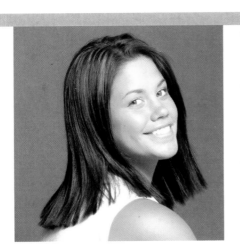

If you measured Yang Moderate or 6 on the Element Barometer, indicating too much Fire in your personality, add Earth to control the Fire. I recommend introducing the Earth element into either the cut or the color, but not both. Earth can stop the Fire or keep it under control depending upon how much is added. Earth will diminish the flames of the Fire.

Haircut to Harmonize Fire/Earth 6

Harmonize with Earth with a blunt style but cut into it to smooth out any overly textured pieces in the haircut. Keep it a natural and clean style while still creating an expressive look. The key is not to be too subtle or it will diminish the spirit of the Fire. I recommend that you select either an Earth cut or color, but not both. Refer to Chapter 11: Hairstyling for Your Body Type, Face Shape, and Facial Features for the best cut for you.

Hair color to Harmonize Fire/Earth 6

Harmonize with Earth by keeping highlighted tones in the same family. Refer to Chapter 11: Hairstyling for Your Body Type, Face Shape, and Facial Features for highlighting placement and techniques. Earth highlighting techniques are more natural and not as obvious as Fire. With Earth highlighting, it should look like sun-kissed streaks.

Balance Fire/Earth 8

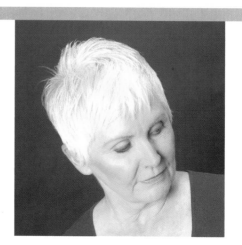

On the Element Barometer, a score of Yang Extreme 8 indicates that you have too much Fire present. I add the Water element to calm the Fire. Fire can be spiraling out of control so I add Water to dampen or harness the energy. Whenever I have a Yang 8 in my chair, I always make recommendations for them to add calm into their lives. Yang Fire types might be more receptive to yoga than meditating. These types need more than a haircut, color, and makeup to bring balance to their lives. I recommend a look on the outside that will definitely have more chic than chaos. It is up to the individual to bring the amount of serenity needed for balance.

Haircut to Balance Fire/Earth 8

Balance with Water by adding texture to the ends for a more chic style. Bring a sense of sensuality to the cut by following Water cutting techniques. Refer to Chapter 11: Hairstyling for Your Body Type, Face Shape, and Facial Features for the best cut. A Water cut will have a flirty look. There will be enough texture to satisfy the creative expression of Fire while harnessing the explosive cuts associated with Fire.

Hair color to Balance Fire/Earth 8

Refer to Water highlighting techniques as well as Chapter 12: Skin Tone and Hair Color. The Water highlighting techniques can have one to three colors for depth. You can use two to seven pieces per pickup. For Fire/Earth, I would recommend two to four pieces and apply in a back-to-back foiling with a brick pattern. You have more color selection with Water than with any other element except Fire. If you are a level five, you can select colors from any level one through ten according to your skin tone.

Fire/Metal

As the tag readily suggests, the Fire/Metal person merges intense curiosity with intense resolve. This resolved, passionate type will never be taken for a compliant wallflower. When balanced, these people are formidable: their passion is driven by a methodical, orderly approach. Fire/Metal types often express Fire in their appearance and Metal in their home, lifestyle, or career. They are extremely detail-oriented and organized in decorating their homes or office, but they will add a creative expression not found in Metal/Metal. Their sense

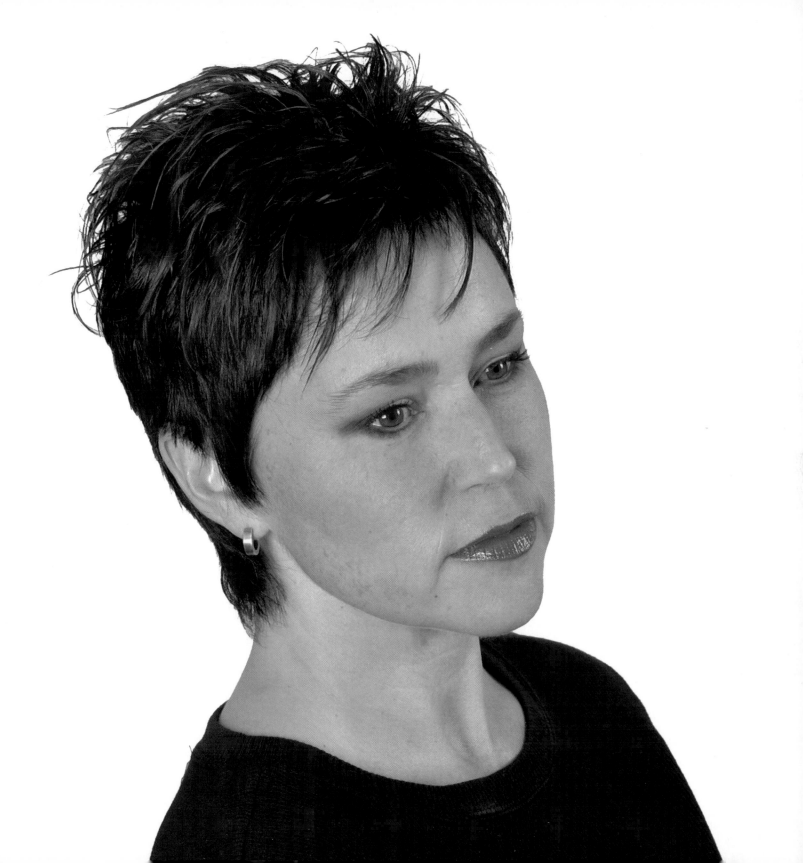

of order does not dampen their artistic expression, but gives it more boundaries. They are willing to wear the latest fad in clothing, accessories, haircut/color, or makeup, but not all at once. They usually have a strong sense of fashion and are willing to try new looks. They will discard them just as quickly if the look does not satisfy their Metal traits. One of our senior managers is a Fire/Metal. She has worked for us part-time for twelve years. She is a department manager for the county so her career requires her to look professional. In her career, she will wear a business suit with a splash of color in her scarf, hat, blouse, shoes, purse, or jewelry. I usually give her a Fire haircut as she loves to change her look with almost every appointment. Her hair color has covered the wide range available to her skin tone. She is very confident with her seemingly conflicting elements. Her office and home are tasteful, colorful, and very Zen. She epitomizes the Fire/Metal 4 as she is balanced and confident to welcome changes in her life.

Persistency and persuasiveness are common traits of Fire/Metal people. They tend to cut to the chase, both in their thought processes and dealings with others. This clarity can be inspiring for others and often places these people in leadership positions or as coveted mates.

Fire/Metal types are excellent in business endeavors especially if they are balanced. They have the creativity and passion of the Fire element along with the discipline, organization, and determination of the Metal element.

Harmonize Fire/Metal 2

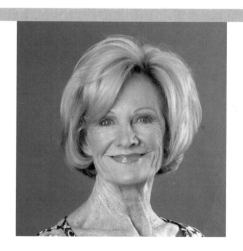

If you measured Yin Extreme or 2 on the Element Barometer, add more expression and feed the Fire. I recommend taking sacred steps to bringing this change by using the Wood element to harmonize the cut and color. Wood will add more movement and encourage the Fire to become more expressive. When I use a Wood cut and/or color, I mix the Wood and Fire colors for makeup by using Wood eye shadow and Fire lipstick.

Haircut to Harmonize Fire/Metal 2
Harmonize with Wood by creating a tousled style with uneven pieces in a random pattern throughout the haircut. Even though the cut will have a lot of texture, it will be contained with a style that will satisfy both the Fire and the Metal elements. Refer to Chapter 11: Hairstyling for Your Body Type, Face Shape, and Facial Features for the best haircut.

Hair color to Harmonize Fire/Metal 2

Harmonize with Wood by adding two to three different colors according to your skin tone and hair color level. If you are a level six, you could select a color from levels four through nine. I recommend using two to three different colors that are close in color. You are striving for a color-on-color effect. Use Wood highlighting techniques which are two to four pieces per pickup. This will give more definition to the highlights. Refer to the chapter on face shape for highlight placement.

Enhance Fire/Metal 4

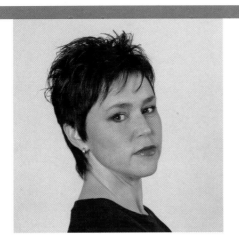

If you measured Yin Moderate or 4 on the Element Barometer, you need to add more Fire. Since the Metal element demands more structure, the Fire will need to be controlled in the cuts and colors. You are not limited in the ways you can add Fire to your life. If your profession demands a more traditional appearance, you may want to release your Fire with your hobbies or by painting your room at home with a splash of color. You must provide an outlet for the Fire whether it is in your lifestyle, artistic endeavors, or dress outside of work. You want to encourage the passion and creativity. Accessories and makeup also provide temporary changes in your appearance.

Haircut to Enhance Fire/Metal 4

Enhance with Fire for a disconnected cut with a pattern of organized chaos. For a short haircut according to your face shape and facial features, you can wear very short cropped hair leaving short spiky pieces around the frame of your face. Refer to Chapter 11: Hairstyling for Your Body Type, Face Shape, and Facial Features for the best length and cut. For more length, I use channeling to add texture and volume.

Hair color to Enhance Fire/Metal 4

Keep your color bold and use two to four different colors to create a Van Gogh feeling. Make the color very expressive using solid colors. With the Fire element, the only limits to your selection of colors or highlighting techniques are your skin tone and natural hair level. Remember that you can wear any color as long as it matches your skin. If you are porcelain, olive, or ebony, these are cool skin tones and would require a cool hair color. If you chose to be blonde, you would want a cool blonde—ash or platinum. If you have a milky, honey, or ruby skin tone, you would want to be a golden or strawberry blonde.

Harmonize Fire/Metal 6

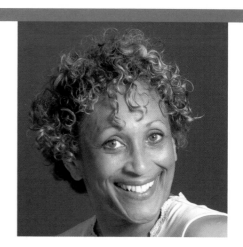

If you measured Yang Moderate or 6 on the Element Barometer, I recommend calming the Fire by adding Earth. Fire creates Earth and Earth creates Metal so Earth is an excellent choice to slow down the Fire and calm the Metal. I recommend the Fire/Metal types add some Earth element to their home environment and/or lifestyle. Earth element types are nurturing and love the warmth of creating in a natural environment free from stress. You want to calm the hectic traits of the Fire element while freeing the confinements of the Metal element. I want to warn you that you will not want to embrace an Earth cut, color, and makeup all at once. I recommend mixing Earth colors and techniques with Fire to suppress the Fire but free up the Metal.

Haircut to Harmonize Fire/Metal 6

Harmonize with Earth by adding texture only to support the hairstyle. Tone the Fire element by creating a more natural look while honoring your Fire element. You don't want to destroy or stop the Fire, only diminish its blaze. Refer to Chapter 11, which discusses face shapes and facial features, for the best styles and lengths for you.

Hair color to Harmonize Fire/Metal 6

Harmonize with Earth by keeping a natural look with the color. Think of how the sun naturally lightens your hair ever so lightly in the summer. I recommend using Earth highlighting techniques and using Earth colors for the color levels. If your hair level is seven, you may select colors from levels five through nine. For highlights, use four to six pieces per pickup for a more natural look. Refer to Chapter 12: Skin Tone and Hair Color for the right colors for you.

Balance Fire/Metal 8

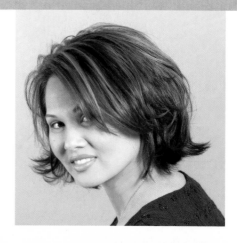

If you measured Yang Extreme or 8 on the Element Barometer, your Fire element and Metal element are in conflict and too strong. This is disruptive as you are exhibiting the extreme traits of both elements. Fire is too hectic and intense while Metal is too unyielding. While the Fire/Metal combination can be dynamite, it can also be destructive if not balanced. Fire types can destroy themselves if not calmed and Metal types can be so uptight that it damages their health. Water is a perfect addition in any aspect of their lives. I recommend reading, meditating, enjoying the performing arts, or visiting a museum. Water clothing and accessories are a perfect way to balance this type also.

Haircut to Balance Fire/Metal 8

Balance with Water by creating a chic, trendy, sassy style according to face shape and facial features (see Chapter 11: Hairstyling for Your Body Type, Face Shape, and Facial Features). Water types are very fashionable, which the Metal type loves, but they also have that kick the Fire craves. Water cuts will have that kick, or extra something, that makes you turn around for a second look or remember how great the person looked.

Hair color to Balance Fire/Metal 8

With Water you can select from a wide variety of colors depending on your element and skin tone. Keep the style chic by adding Water highlighting techniques such as slices according to your face shape and features to keep a flirty look. See Chapter 12: Skin Tone and Hair Color.

Fire/Water

Those with the duality of Fire and Water are often a study in contradictions and ambiguity. The fluidity and flexibility of their Water traits may undermine their passion and optimism. This contradiction of traits sometimes suggests a fickleness or lack of resolve. Like a meandering stream, they tend to shift course when encountering complications. At the same time, they can adapt to a variety of people and circumstances, shifting to meet the moment.

When in balance, Fire/Water types are a formidable opponent or business associate. The creativity and passion of Fire becomes extremely productive when the Water element provides the thirst for knowledge and background that is vital for new endeavors or ventures to succeed. A great friend of mine provides insight to this combination. In his chosen profession, I can think of no one more passionate about his work and more creative in developing new techniques to achieve results. This Fire/Water type is always willing to try new methods to reach his goal. He uses Fire in his passion and creativity mixed with his love of meditation and knowledge to achieve success not only in reaching goals, but also in bringing his associates into the process. That, to me, is truly Fire/Water in balance.

The Fire element reacts to situations immediately and the Water element likes to meditate and weigh each bit of information. When in balance, the combination is very creative and forward-thinking. It is an awesome combination for success. You welcome new fashions and new styles and wear them with ease.

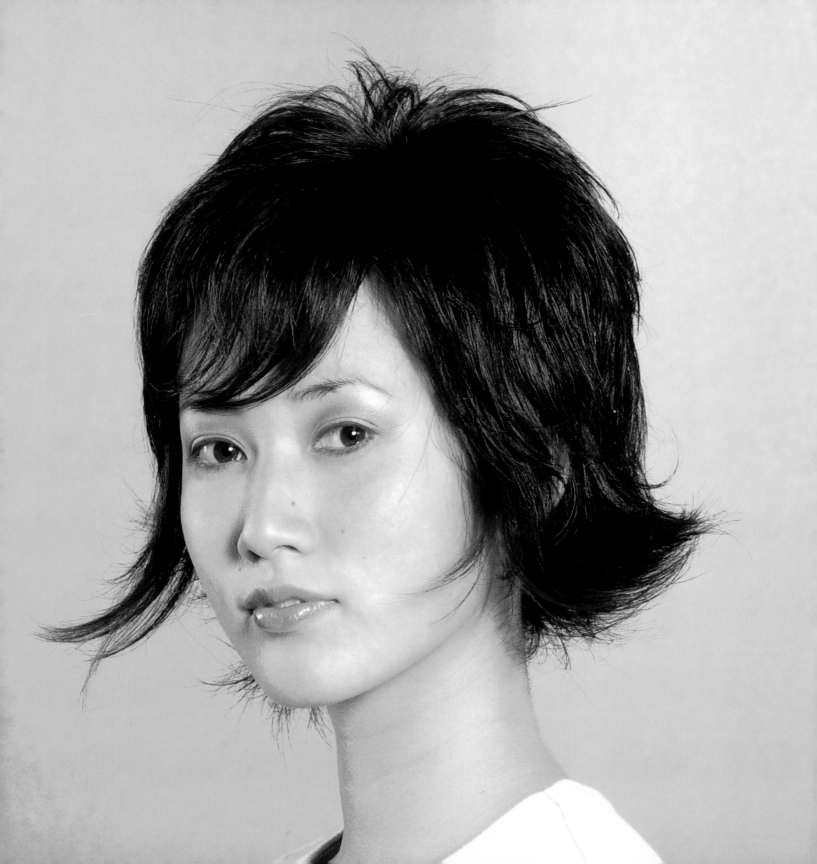

Harmonize Fire/Water 2

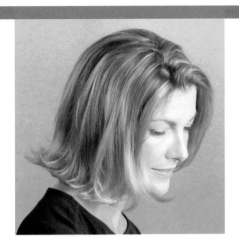

If you scored Yin Extreme or 2 on the Element Barometer, use Wood element to feed the Fire and allow for more expression in your life and fashion. I suggest that you use Wood cutting and coloring techniques. I recommend that you become involved with an activity or hobby that requires you to be outdoors.

Haircut to Harmonize Fire/Water 2

Harmonize with Wood by creating a tousled, active, shorter cut. If you desire to keep your hair longer, have longer layers to let the hair flow and add movement. Refer to Chapter 11: Hairstyling for Your Body Type, Face Shape, and Facial Features for the best cuts. Curly hair is great for this tousled look. Hair should not have a structured or "set" look. Strive for a casual style.

Hair color to Harmonize Fire/Water 2

Use Wood highlighting techniques. If your hair is curly, you would use two to three pieces per pickup with your weave. You need to be able to see the color amidst the curls. Select color from the lower levels on the color chart. For example, if your hair is a level six, you can select from colors level three, four, or five. This will give you richer, deeper color or lowlights. Chapter 12 will refer you to the right colors for you.

Enhance Fire/Water 4

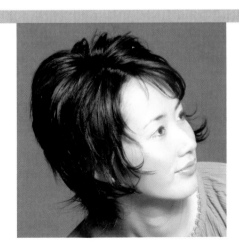

If you measured Yin Moderate or 4 on the Element Barometer, you will need to add more Fire to bring out the unexpressed Fire inside. I recommend adding either a Fire haircut or Fire color. If you are willing to accept a drastic change in your appearance, a Fire cut and color might be just the look you need to release your creative expression. With a Fire/Water type, you can wear a Fire haircut, Fire highlights, and Water color. You need to feel comfortable with the options available to you.

Haircut to Enhance Fire/Water 4

Enhance Fire with a disconnected, edgy, rebellious, but not bold cut. You set the limits as your type is one that loves the latest looks and can wear them with ease. Refer to Chapter 11: Hairstyling for Your Body Type, Face Shape, and Facial Features for the best cut for you. Your adventurous spirit can serve as your guide.

Hair color to Enhance Fire/Water 4

Be daring in your selection of highlighting techniques. For your color, refer to the chapter on skin tones and element colors. Fire has no boundaries on color except for skin tone. Once you have determined your skin tone, select colors from the correct element and skin tone information. I suggest tones of color that do not blend together, but that stand out from one another. In other words, do not select subtle tone-on-tone colors. For highlighting, the back-to-back slicing will add bold colors.

Harmonize Fire/Water 6

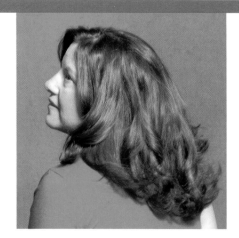

If you scored Yang Moderate or 6 on the Element Barometer, use Earth to subdue the excess Fire. Fire creates Earth; however, adding Earth to Fire will slow it down just as with the Water element. Earth will stop Water or control it. It is important when using the Earth element to harmonize so that you don't use too much and diminish the passion and excitement of the Fire element. Harmonizing the cut and color with Earth will bring a more natural look to your style. You would want to select either an Earth cut or color but not both.

Haircut to Harmonize Fire/Water 6

Harmonize with Earth by keeping simple, soft lines in your style. Be careful to keep some movement and texture while creating a natural style. Refer to Chapter 11: Hairstyling for Your Body Type, Face Shape, and Facial Features for the best cut.

Hair color to Harmonize Fire/Water 6

Harmonize with Earth by referring to the chapter on skin tones and element colors. Select colors either two levels down or two levels up. If you were a level seven, you could wear level five or six, or eight or nine. Highlighting techniques would be more natural—like the sun streaking. Use four to six pieces per pickup for a natural look. Check the chapter on face shapes for highlighting techniques and placement for your face shape and element.

Balance Fire/Water 8

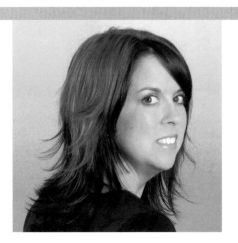

If you scored Yang Extreme or 8 on the Element Barometer, balance with the Water element. Water element calms Fire if added in moderation. Since the Fire/Water type has Water as its second element, you can be expressive and creative with Water colors and techniques. Water will add a chic look to the explosive extreme Fire element. Too much Water will put out the Fire, so you will want to add either a Water cut or Water color, but not both. I recommend that the Water element be introduced in clothing, lifestyle, accessories, or hobby as well. This will add a new dimension of calm to the Fire element.

Haircut to Balance Fire/Water 8

Balance with Water by creating a sassy, flirty, out-of-the-box cut that is chic but strong. Make sure the cut and style are not spiky or disconnected. Refer to Chapter 11: Hairstyling for Your Body Type, Face Shape, and Facial Features for the best cut.

Hair color to Balance Fire/Water 8

Use the Water color chart found in Chapter 12: Skin Tone and Hair Color for your skin tone and hair level. With Water, you can try more colors and achieve the expression you want. If you are a natural level four, you can select colors from levels zero through nine. Be certain to determine if your skin tone is cool or warm. Porcelain, Olive, and Ebony are the cool tones and require that you select cool colors. Milky, Honey, and Ruby are warm tones. Skin tones may change with exposure to the sun. Follow the guidelines in the chapter for determining your skin tone. For highlighting techniques, you can be creative with Water techniques. Select back-to-back, brick, or Van Gogh techniques. Be sure to consider your face shape when placing highlights for the best results. This information is found in Chapter 11: Hairstyling for Your Body Type, Face Shape, and Facial Features.

Fire/Wood

The Fire/Wood person is quick to assess a situation and just as quick to have a response. Instead of an indifference to the nuances of the circumstances, Fire/Wood types hunger for solutions and results. This focus on the results, and single-mindedness for resolve, sometimes makes Fire/Woods appear dogmatic and inflexible.

Fire/Wood people are often the best advocates for an unorthodox position. Once they've accepted a concept, they're apt to commit fully to it and focus on doing anything necessary to make it happen.

Wood feeds Fire and, if left without restraint, Fire can consume itself. Fire/Wood people benefit from gentle guidance and supportive direction. Fire/Wood types are usually fun and outgoing. They draw people to them with their passion and love of fun. They are people watchers by nature. They never meet a stranger and use each encounter to gain information. They know the life history of their taxi driver and the man who shines their shoes. Many Fire/Wood types have gotten their post-secondary education from the people they spend time with. They ask questions to seek information and will shamelessly spend hours with others seeking their views on a myriad of subjects.

It is imperative that Fire/Wood types stay focused or they can get out of hand. They have a hard time making a decision as they have received so many different ideas. Their opinions may change from day to day, depending on any new information they receive. This is not to say that they have no ideas of their own; I believe they are seekers of information and utilize the information to create new techniques and skills. Fire/Wood types are passionate about their work and hobbies. They seek hobbies or activities that involve others as they prefer the company of others. These are the types that a hostess loves to have at any function. They are charismatic and the darling of any crowd.

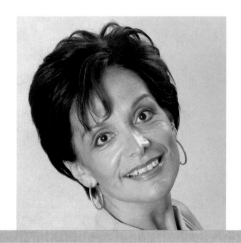

In fashion, they prefer dramatic colors and styles that set them apart. For exercise, they will usually go to the extreme and may follow each fad diet until the next one comes along.

Harmonize Fire/Wood 2

If you measured Yin Extreme or 2 on the Element Barometer, harmonize your cut or color with Wood. Remember Wood feeds Fire, so don't add too much or it will cause the Fire to be out of control. I recommend either a Wood cut and Fire color or Fire cut and Wood color.

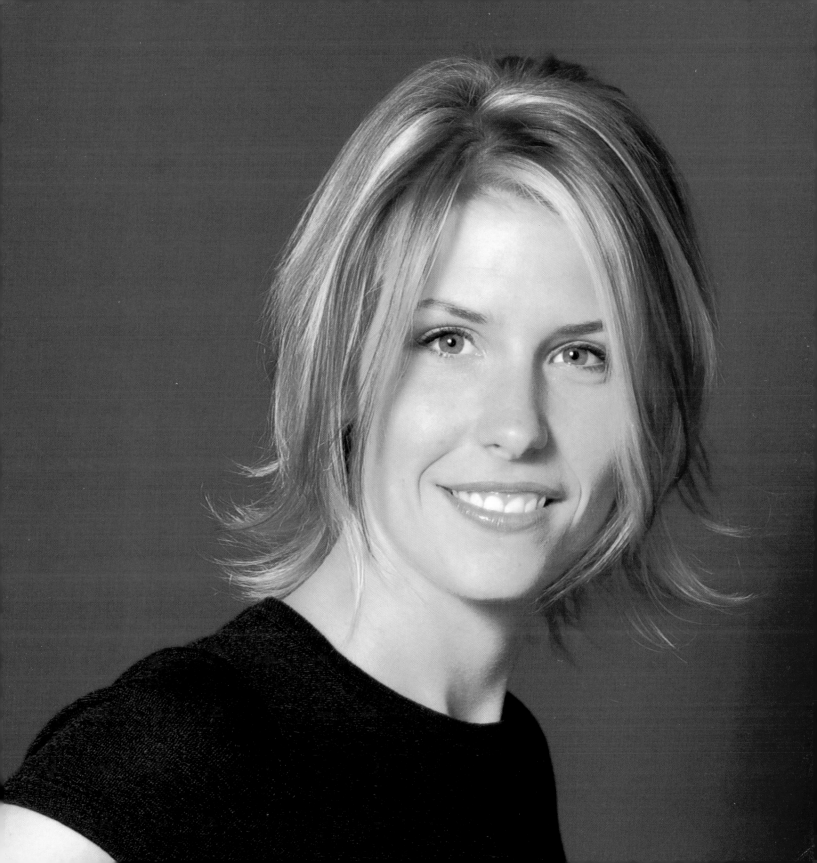

Haircut to Harmonize Fire/Wood 2

Harmonize with Wood to create a tousled, short, and sporty cut. You want hair that looks wind-blown or that has lots of movement. If you select to keep your hair longer, wear long full layers that will give you the movement needed without creating a thinner longer layer at the bottom. Refer to Chapter 11: Hairstyling for Your Body Type, Face Shape, and Facial Features for the best cut.

Hair color to Harmonize Fire/Wood 2

Harmonize with Wood by using deeper, richer colors for all over color. Refer to Chapter 12: Skin Tone and Hair Color for the range of colors available to you. If you are a natural level five, I would suggest that you select tones from level three or four for deeper colors. Use Chapter 11: Hairstyling for Your Body Type, Face Shape, and Facial Features for highlighting techniques and highlight placement.

Enhance Fire/Wood 4

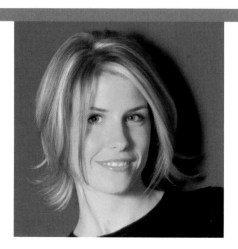

If you measure Yin Moderate or 4 on the Element Barometer, you need to add more Fire to your appearance. I balance the Fire by mixing a Wood color or makeup. Enhance the Fire in order to express a more dramatic look in your appearance.

Haircut to Enhance Fire/Wood 4

Enhance with Fire by adding texture to create uneven pieces for movement with styling. Since Wood feeds Fire, you can be more daring when you are a Fire/Wood. Refer to Chapter 11: Hairstyling for Your Body Type, Face Shape, and Facial Features for the best cut. If you have curly hair, I use artichoke cutting techniques to give a free flowing look without weighing down the style.

Hair color to Enhance Fire/Wood 4

Enhance with Fire techniques which allow you to be very creative. Select colors from the chapter on skin tone and element colors. The only boundary for Fire element is skin tone. Make certain that you select a color according to your skin tone in the Fire section. Refer to the chapter on face shape and highlighting techniques for highlight placement. You can be as daring as you want when selecting color or techniques.

Harmonize Fire/Wood 6

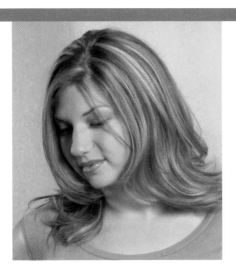

If you measure Yang Moderate or 6 on the Element Barometer, you need to add Earth to calm the Fire. By adding Earth slowly, you diminish the flame without extinguishing it. Since Wood balances or stops Earth, be careful to add Earth influences in your cut or color, but not both. You might want to introduce Earth influences in your lifestyle, accessories, or clothing to harmonize Fire/Wood. Fire and Wood both tend to be aggressive or outgoing, moving forward. If the movement is too fast, Earth will slow them down.

Haircut to Harmonize Fire/Wood 6

Harmonize with Earth by adding medium length layers or soft layers if the style is shorter. Refer to Chapter 11: Hairstyling for Your Body Type, Face Shape, and Facial Features for the best cut. Earth element styles are more natural and blunt cut. I recommend adjusting the style by adding softness and movement.

Hair color to Harmonize Fire/Wood 6

Harmonize with Earth with softer colors or tone on tone Earth highlights. Refer to Chapter 12: Skin Tone and Hair Color for the color selection. You will not want a dramatic look in your color but rather a more natural look. Look at Chapter 11: Hairstyling for Your Body Type, Face Shape, and Facial Features for highlighting techniques and highlighting placement.

Balance Fire/Wood 8

If you measure Yang Extreme or 8 on the Element Barometer, you need to add Water to balance the overabundance of Fire. Too much Water will extinguish Fire. Adding the right amount of Water will produce steam or make the Fire more productive. I recommend using either a Water cut or color to balance the look. I also suggest that you add the Water element to your lifestyle by meditating or reflecting on your life. Fire/Wood types are outgoing and, when Yang Extreme, need to slow down and think before moving ahead so rapidly.

Haircut to Balance Fire/Wood 8

Balance with Water for a flirty, kicky, feminine approach to a sensual look. Refer to Chapter 11: Hairstyling for Your Body Type, Face Shape, and Facial Features for the best cut. Regardless of your hair texture or the length you select for your hair, the overall look must be feminine and sassy.

Hair color to Balance Fire/Wood 8

Balance with Water using bolder colors found in Chapter 12: Skin Tone and Hair Color. Since you are able to select colors from a wide range according to the chart, be creative in your use of colors. If you are a natural level seven, you may select colors from levels three through twelve. Refer to Chapter 11: Hair-styling for Your Body Type, Face Shape, and Facial Features for highlighting techniques and placement.

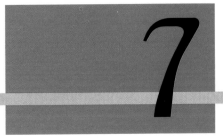

7 Earth Element

An Earth personality exudes serenity and a genuine concern for others. Earth's basic nature is to protect and sustain life. Earth types are the foundation of friendships, homes, organizations, and businesses. They are givers and will take on others' problems until their energy is depleted. Wherever there is someone in need or who has a problem to be solved, the Earth type will be the first to make time. It is difficult for Earth types to receive compliments or gifts gracefully—they feel unworthy. Earth personalities are motherly and nurturing. They can easily be taken advantage of, as they are trusting of others. They are also totally trustworthy in any relationship.

Earth personalities tend to be self-reliant, independent, practical, and have the aptitude to work hard and patiently build their fortune. They are efficient managers of resources and gravitate toward down-to-earth activities. The positive mental states associated with Earth are truthfulness, trustworthiness, patience, sympathy, compassion, firmness, and determination. Earth personalities tend to be responsive, steadfast, and supportive, while at the same time emotionally reserved and shy.

Earth people tend to avoid risk, and their practical help to others usually includes risk-avoidance. Hand-in-hand with this distaste for risk is the hunger for security and safety. Just as Earth types gravitate toward safety, these personalities also tend to make others feel protected and nurtured. Left to their own devices, Earth personalities will embrace the familiar and be content with consistency. They are often more comfortable in a behind-the-scenes role and serve as excellent advisors to the designated leader.

Earth types prefer to fade into the background and will resist being the center of attention. Their preferred style is neither flashy nor the latest fashion. Although their appearance is never untidy, they prefer comfort and clean, simple lines in their clothing. Earth types look for a natural, low-key approach to their makeup, accessories, clothing, and hair. Their appearance is not the first thing you notice about an Earth type but rather their genuine warmth and focus. Others gravitate towards Earth types.

Earth types must be replenished by finding time for themselves. Think of soil being depleted after a harvest and never receiving any of the fertilizers or minerals needed for replenishment. From time to time, Earth types need to splurge on luxury items and be pampered—whether at home or in a spa—in order to nourish their souls. Sometimes it is difficult for Earth types to move forward into the future and think about goal setting. It is easy for them to get stuck in the present and become bogged down by minute details and problems.

Protecting the environment is usually a concern and project for Earth types. They are quick to organize clean-up days at the beach or park. They are also very involved in organizations and charities for children and animals. Earth types make excellent caretakers for children, the elderly, or the ill. It is this trait of compassion that they take into any career and that makes them invaluable.

Earth persons are typically loyal, reliable, and persistent. When committed to a task, their patience and persistence will enable them to see it through to completion. If you have an Earth person for a friend, you are indeed lucky. The Earth type is always there for you and is willing to cancel any previous appointment if you need someone to lean on. The Earth personality will listen as long as you need. They are extremely supportive of others and non-judgmental. They are in the Now and are there for you.

Within each element, Yin and Yang energies exist. On the Element Barometer, I have listed characteristics that will assist you in knowing whether you need to enhance, harmonize, or balance the element. If the Earth element is hidden or Yin Extreme 2, you need to add the Fire element to encourage more spark. When the Yin is Moderate 4, you need to enhance the Earth. If the Yang is Moderate 6, you need to add the Metal element for structure. When the Earth element is too extreme Yang 8, I recommend using Wood to stabilize.

The intensity of Earth that we express can be compared to the different types of earth. Earth that is unstable can create a landslide and cause havoc if not stabilized. In California, people have a tendency to build homes on cliffs or on unstable land in order to capture a spectacular view. It is critical to stabilize such land with wood piers for support or balance. People who have too much Earth become too isolated and unwilling to accept new ideas. That is similar to a Yang Extreme 8 on the Element Barometer. A Yang Moderate 6 would be similar to blowing topsoil or sand dunes that need to be contained by plants, fences, or structures placed strategically to stop erosion. A person who is a Yang Moderate 6 would need organization and discipline for their Earth element to create structure. A Yin Moderate 4 needs to have rich topsoil added to enhance its fertile soil. Earth types who are Moderate 4 need to receive caring and nurturing to feed their souls. Earth that is barren or depleted must receive fertilizer and minerals in order to become productive again. Fire produces ashes, which add minerals to the soil; this is used to generate new earth. A Yin Extreme 2 type needs to add Fire to add spark or energy to their lives as they need the rejuvenation and added minerals to bring harmony and production.

Using Feng Shui principles designed to bring balance or create a flow of good Chi, I take into consideration not only your haircut, hair color, makeup, body type, and face shape, but also your hobbies, your lifestyle, your exercise patterns, meditation, clothing, and accessories. All of these things affect you and the image you portray. When I prescribe the look that will best reflect how you perceive yourself, I also make recommendations to other factors that influence your life. Some of the recommendations or changes will be evident almost immediately such as haircut, hair color, and makeup. The other changes will involve more participation and will evolve as you are the one in charge of implementing that part of your life. The amount of change will depend upon your dedication.

Makeup for the Earth Element

Although applying makeup might not be an important part of your routine, I recommend adding soft natural colors to enhance your natural beauty. Select the colors recommended for your skin tone. You may usually only wear lipstick or eye shadow. Keeping with the colors recommended for Earth, you should feel comfortable wearing both and still have an understated look.

Porcelain

Put a light dusting of mauve to pink on eyelids and use soft pink, sheer lip gloss.

Milky

Try soft peach and ivory on eyelids, with nude lips.

Honey

Use soft browns on lids and soft nude to brown on lips.

Olive

You'll do well with soft mauve sheer shadow using a light touch or airbrush application and lips in mauve *au natural* shades.

Ebony

Try a brown shadow with a brown-brick nude lip color.

Ruby

Go with natural ivory or brown eye shadow and nude lips.

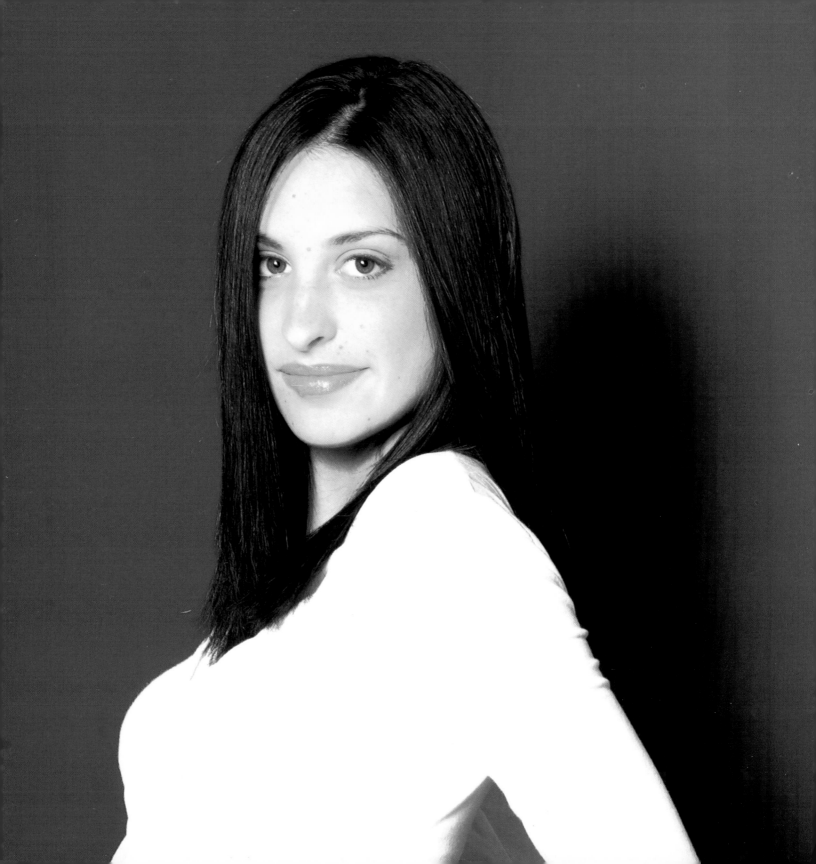

Earth/Fire

The Earth/Fire combo may appear a tough nut to crack. The Fire component tends to inspire insightful approaches for this otherwise stay-the-course, grounded person. While naturally reserved and down-to-earth, the Earth/Fire person often appears to blossom around the familiar, showing a more gregarious side in private among trusted allies. In their role as an advisor, they often display creative brilliance in crafting solutions in furtherance of their supporting role. The Earth's natural loyalty becomes fiercer when combined with Fire.

As a business owner, the Earth/Fire is concerned with creating a warm environment for employees and clients/customers. Their gracious demeanor means that you are never just a number, but the Earth/Fire type knows and remembers you. In fact, if you are in need of an item, an Earth/Fire type will special order it for you and see that you have it on time. This is extraordinary in most business arenas and certainly sets them apart. If Earth/Fire types are wise, they will insist on hiring Metal element types for their accounting and bookkeeping needs as discipline and details are Metal's forte.

The Earth/Fire enjoys sharing gifts from the garden or kitchen. The Earth/Fire types pay attention to the smallest details from the wrapping to the note that accompanies the gift. They are great hostesses and their party invitations are treasured. As a teacher, they offer the best of both worlds. They are caring and nurturing while possessing that creative energy that makes you want to learn and listen to what they are saying. As artists, their creative expressions are warm and colorful.

Harmonize Earth/Fire 2

If you measured Yin Extreme or 2 on the Element Barometer, this indicates that even though you give and give, it may be depleting your energy. You sacrifice for others and are not able to gauge when enough is enough. You need to add Fire to add more energy. Fire creates Earth so Fire energy will replenish the Earth. Fire types are creative and expressive in their look and very passionate in their actions. By adding Fire to the Earth/Fire types, you will add expression and passion to their causes and beliefs. I recommend the Earth/Fire type become active in some form of exercise, yoga, or outdoor activity. Fire will inspire and serve as a catalyst for creativity within the Earth element. I recommend selecting one or two of the three choices below.

Haircut to Harmonize Earth/Fire 2

Harmonize with Fire by adding more texture throughout the haircut. One example for a short haircut would be a pixie cut with lots of pieces around the face and an uneven neck line. You want to add interest to the haircut by creating texture without disarray. A Fire haircut for longer hair would involve cutting uneven pieces throughout. If you are creating layers, it is important the layers not be too thin and wispy. Creating a Fire haircut for curly hair demands the texture of the hair be considered. Cutting uneven pieces in extremely curly hair will add an artichoke look, creating volume and bounce. Refer to Chapter 11: Hairstyling for Your Body Type, Face Shape, and Facial Features for the best cut.

Hair color to Harmonize Earth/Fire 2

Harmonize by using the highlighting techniques found Chapter 11: Hairstyling for Your Body Type, Face Shape, and Facial Features. I recommend using back-to-back slices for a more artistic bold look. You are not striving for subtle or natural highlights, but rather highlights that demand to be noticed. Depending on your natural hair color level, you may refer to Chapter 12: Skin Tone and Hair Color for the best color. You decide how bold you want to be—always be respectful of your Earth type.

Enhance Earth/Fire 4

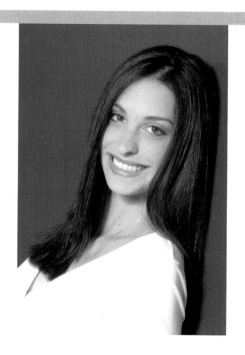

If you measured Yin Moderate or 4 on the Element Barometer, this signifies that you need to enhance your Earth by adding more Earth. Your Earth element has been depleted and you may be feeling overwhelmed by your responsibilities and outside influences. It may be time to get back to the basics in your appearance. By adding an Earth haircut, color, and/or makeup, you will be creating a more natural look.

Haircut to Enhance Earth/Fire 4

Enhance with Earth for a blunt cut to lose any disconnected or uneven pieces in the previous haircut. Keep the cut and style very natural with clean lines. Add texture for soft movement. Creating an Earth cut for curly hair means letting it fall naturally and unrestricted. Refer to Chapter 11: Hairstyling for Your Body Type, Face Shape, and Facial Features for the best haircut.

Hair color to Enhance Earth/Fire 4

Enhance the color by referring to Chapter 12: Skin Tone and Hair Color. With Earth colors, if you are a level six, you may select colors from levels four or five, or seven or eight. Refer to Chapter 11: Hairstyling for Your Body Type, Face Shape, and Facial Features for highlighting techniques and placement. Since you are an Earth/Fire, I recommend using four to five pieces per pickup for a bolder look.

Harmonize Earth/Fire 6

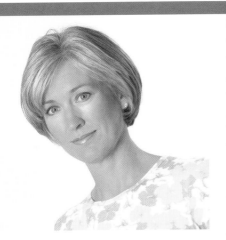

If you measured Yang Moderate or 6 on the Element Barometer, you have too much Earth in your personality. Too much Earth renders the Earth/Fire element unable to function at its highest level. You will need to add Metal to bring order and efficiency to your lifestyle. A Metal person is more focused and moves quickly to bring action to goals. Fashion for Earth types is usually an afterthought as they prefer styles that do not take too much time. When an Earth/Fire type needs a more professional look, I recommend adding a classic Metal haircut or color. It would be too restrictive to have a Metal haircut, color, and makeup all at the same time, but one addition will harmonize you.

Haircut to Harmonize Earth/Fire 6

Harmonize with Metal by keeping the style one length and softening the ends. When you think about Metal cuts, think of a classic bob that never goes out of style. Refer to Chapter 11: Hairstyling for Your Body Type, Face Shape, and Facial Features for the best haircut. If you select a mid-length haircut, find the perfect length based on your face shape. For a short haircut, the shortest point will usually be mid-way between your cheekbone and jawline. If your hair is curly, you can still wear a bob or classic style.

Hair color to Harmonize Earth/Fire 6

Harmonize with Metal by kicking the color up one notch or by using Metal highlighting and colors. Metal highlighting techniques are more refined and the color selection blends with the overall color. In other words, you would not want contrasting colors or a sharp definition between the colors as you might find with Fire color and highlighting. Refer to Chapter 11: Hairstyling for Your Body Type, Face Shape, and Facial Features for highlighting techniques, application, and placement. Select your color from the chapter on Skin tone and Elements. If you are a natural level seven, you can select colors from levels four through eleven. This presents a wide choice and will depend on your skin tone and how comfortable you are with change.

Balance Earth/Fire 8

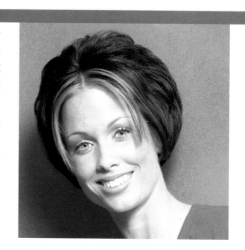

If you measure Yang Extreme or 8 on the Element Barometer, your Earth element has you stuck in the present. You can't focus on new ideas or the future. It is time to add some new ideas and new activities to your life. I suggest bringing the Wood element into your lifestyle as well as your look. Wood breaks up Earth and keeps it from becoming too hard. Too much Earth becomes an immovable hill. Earth types can become stubborn and unyielding, which results in a withdrawal from others. By introducing Wood activities and opportunities for a more social environment, the Yang Extreme Earth/Fire type has the chance to make positive changes that will bring you into balance.

Haircut to Balance Earth/Fire 8

Balance with Wood by selecting a style that uses notching or chunking shears for texture. This will add more pizzazz to the cut without causing havoc to the clean no-fuss style. You want to add movement and energy into the cut. Refer to Chapter 11: Hairstyling for Your Body Type, Face Shape, and Facial Features for the best cut. You can certainly be daring with your Wood cut as you have the Fire element influence.

Hair color to Balance Earth/Fire 8

Balance the color with Wood with adding sun-kissed highlights with tone-on-tone colors. Select the color from Chapter 12: Skin Tone and Hair Color. If you are a natural level five, you may select levels three or four, or six through eight. If you select a color from six through eight, you might want to add lowlights for depth. Refer to Chapter 11: Hairstyling for Your Body Type, Face Shape, and Facial Features for highlight placement and techniques. Wood highlighting techniques allow for a sporty look that is achieved with a two to four piece pickup as opposed to a four to six piece pickup with an Earth weave. You will get more color with a Wood highlighting technique.

Earth/Earth

While the Earth element tends to crave security and familiarity, the Earth/Earth person is nearly obsessive about this craving. This tendency may result in predictability and/or close-mindedness. As a result, the Earth/Earth type may get stuck in routines and find it difficult to enjoy new experiences.

The double Earth people push for consistency in all areas of their life. They thirst for long-term commitments, whether in their personal lives or in their career. Because consistency and familiarity are their overriding objectives, they tend to tolerate lesser grievances for the sake of guarding consistency. For the double Earth person, change—whether in hairstyle, career, or personal relationships—can be a very tough pill to swallow. I recommend sacred steps in changing your appearance. A gradual change is more in keeping with the Earth/Earth personality.

An Earth/Earth type excels in a service industry position such as education, social services, clergy, nursing, or medicine. It is the genuine caring and empathy that makes this type so valuable in working with individuals in need. Think of Mother Teresa who devoted her life to caring for dying individuals who lived in the streets and had no one else to hold them as they departed from this earth. Others were comforted by knowing her; her spirit and love made their burdens more bearable. The double Earth will be the one who can become so involved with others' problems that they become physically sick. It is imperative that they receive caring and love from others in order to replenish their emotional and physical state. Earth/Earth types need to seek a release away from people. Reading, gardening, strolling through a park, or enjoying a long bath with lighted candles and soft music are excellent activities for the double Earth. A walk along the ocean or observing spring flowers in the garden are great occasions for an opportunity to enjoy the beauty in Mother Earth.

Harmonize Earth/Earth 2

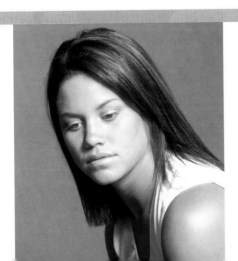

If you measured Yin Extreme or 2 on the Element Barometer, you will need to increase the presence of Fire in your look. The challenge is to know how much Fire to add. You have to know what you are comfortable with adding. If you have had the same haircut and color for a long time, you might want to experiment with adding either a Fire haircut or hair color. If my recommendations for haircut and color don't appeal to you, look at the suggestions under Fire makeup in Chapter 13. The changes do not have to occur at one time but can be added as gradually as you decide. The goal is for you to be in charge of how and when you want to change your appearance.

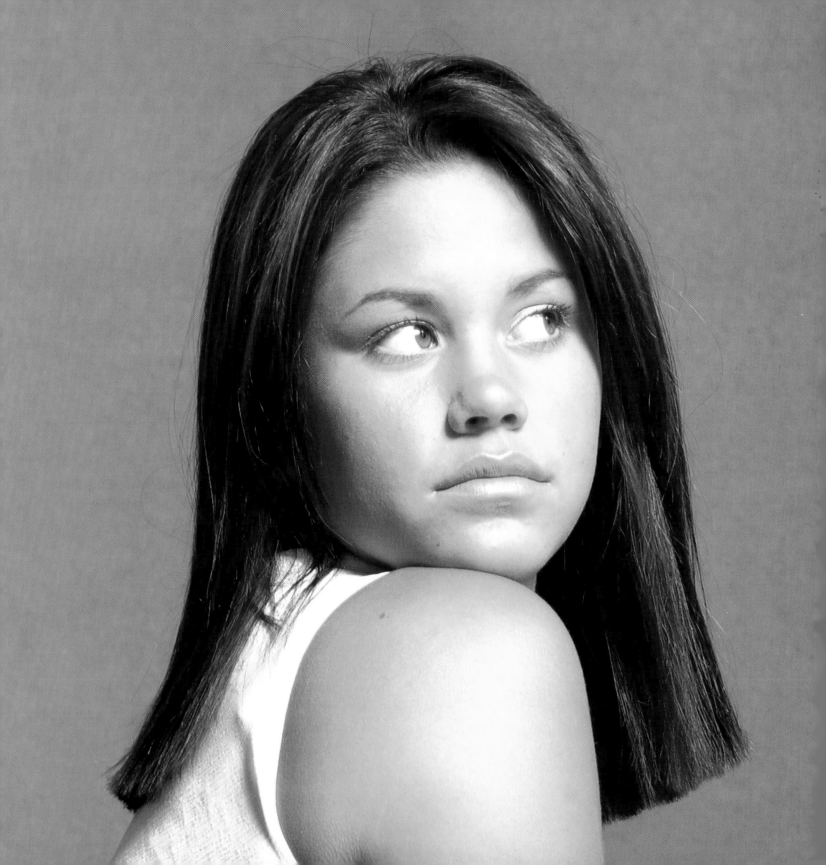

Haircut to Harmonize Earth/Earth 2

Harmonize your cut with Fire by using a razor for texture. You want to create expression and movement in the cut. Earth cuts are usually blunt and/or one length. By cutting into the hair, it moves more freely and isn't weighed down. For longer hair I recommend longer layers that may be either rounded for inward movement or concave for outward expression. With short hair, break up the hair by creating layers. Be subtle, as less is more. Be cautious, as more extensive layering demands that you spend more time styling your hair. Refer to Chapter 11: Hairstyling for Your Body Type, Face Shape, and Facial Features for the best cut. Please keep in mind that you do not want an explosive, bold haircut, but one that has more expression.

Hair color to Harmonize Earth/Earth 2

Harmonize with Fire by referring to Chapter 12: Skin Tone and Hair Color for the range of colors available according to your skin tone. With Fire, the only limitation is your skin tone. It is important not to be too radical in changing your hair color if your elements are Earth/Earth. You might consider using Earth color with Fire highlights. Look Chapter 11: Hairstyling for Your Body Type, Face Shape, and Facial Features for highlight placement and techniques. You don't want to shock, but you do want to add some color and excitement to your hair.

Enhance Earth/Earth 4

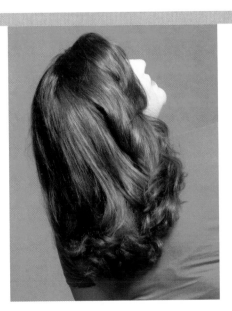

If you measure Yin Moderate or 4 on the Element Barometer, you need to increase the presence of Earth in your look. You need to add enough to boost your Earth element. You may not be honoring the natural, clean lines in your haircut. Earth/Earth types prefer a no-fuss hairstyle that almost takes care of itself. With the addition of Earth element, you want to make certain the look will still be as professional as you need.

Haircut to Enhance Earth/Earth 4

Enhance with Earth by keeping a clean simple line to the cut to create an organic look that flows naturally. A one-length blunt cut is usually the cut of preference for this type. You will not want to create a lot of texture or movement, but rather let the hair hang and move naturally. Regardless of the length of your hair, it should always complement your face shape and facial features. Refer to Chapter 11: Hairstyling for Your Body Type, Face Shape, and Facial Features for the best haircut and the best length.

Hair color to Enhance Earth/Earth 4

Choose colors from Chapter 12: Skin Tone and Hair Color. An Earth type wants to select colors that are more close to your natural level. If you are a natural level four, you could select levels two through six. Refer to Chapter 11: Hairstyling for Your Body Type, Face Shape, and Facial Features for highlighting techniques and placement. Your goal will to achieve color that looks as though nature added the highlights.

Harmonize Earth/Earth 6

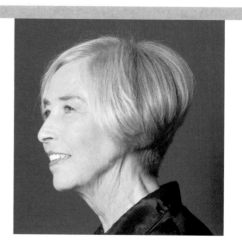

If you measured Yang Moderate or 6 on the Element Barometer, you will add Metal for structure. Yang Moderate 6 means that you have an abundance of Earth element and need to harness the Earth by containing it. Metal element is more focused and concerned with meeting deadlines for any project. Earth element types are not as concerned with timelines as with completing the task in as stress-free a manner as possible. Metal element types have the characteristics that Earth elements desire. This is especially true in the ability to rid their lives of clutter and setting goals that require discipline and organizational skills to achieve. Although Earth/Earth types long for the structure of Metal, they find it much too restrictive and will give up rather than gradually add a little Metal at a time. I recommend that you begin with one aspect of the Metal element. If you are hesitant about making drastic changes, begin with either a Metal haircut, color, highlight, or makeup. You may also wish to plan an evening listening to classical music at home or at the symphony, attending opening night at the theater, or revisiting Shakespeare at your convenience. With Feng Shui, you are the one who decides how and when you wish to make changes. You can change your appearance, hobby, career, or any aspect of your life.

Haircut to Harmonize Earth/Earth 6

Harmonize with Metal by selecting a semi-classic style that uses softening shears for a professional look without sharp edges. If you select a bob for your haircut, you will want to make certain it is not too severe. Refer to Chapter 11: Hairstyling for Your Body Type, Face Shape, and Facial Features for the best haircut and the best length for you.

Hair color to Harmonize Earth/Earth 6

Harmonize the color by using Metal highlighting techniques and/or selecting Metal colors listed in Chapter 12: Skin Tone and Hair Color. The color selection is wider with Metal colors than with Earth colors. If you are a level six, you can select colors from three to nine. This wide range of colors will add more variance for an Earth/Earth. It is vital that you select a color that matches your skin tone. Since most Earth/Earth types are reluctant to make drastic changes in their appearance, I recommend a more gradual change in color and recommend using Metal highlighting techniques that are very precise.

Balance Earth/Earth 8

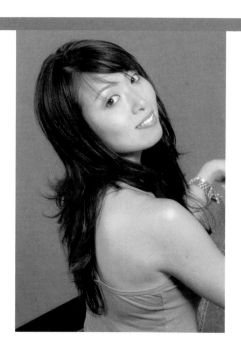

If you measure Yang Extreme or 8 on the Element Barometer, you need to balance with Wood. Wood stabilizes Earth when it is in danger of being out of control. Wood element hairstyles are free flowing with lots of movement. There will be more expression with Wood colors and highlighting techniques. Wood element styles project an active or sporty style, but one that does require some time to achieve. Again, I recommend that you begin your makeover or change gradually and add either a Wood haircut or hair color.

Haircut to Balance Earth/Earth 8
Balance with Wood for an easy to maintain, active tousled style. Refer to Chapter 11: Hairstyling for Your Body Type, Face Shape, and Facial Features for the best cut for you. If you have curly hair, this is the ideal element for you. The tousled look with free flowing curls will have bounce and style with a rounded layer cut or with alternating layers of cutting into the bend of the hair. This method gives the curls more movement and keeps them from being weighed down.

Hair color to Balance Earth/Earth 8
Add deeper rich colors from Chapter 12: Skin Tone and Hair Color. Wood element colors are very close to Earth element color level choices. If you are a natural level seven, with the Wood element you may select levels five through ten. For highlighting techniques refer to Chapter 11: Hairstyling for Your Body Type, Face Shape, and Facial Features for techniques and highlight placement. Using Wood element highlighting techniques from Chapter 12, you will have more separate pieces of color and more color will be obvious.

Earth/Metal

The Earth/Metal person is often a formidable force. Persistence, when coupled with methodical, organized execution, enables Earth/Metal people to work patiently towards their objectives. Earth/Metal's natural empathy for others can be strongly influenced by their clear-thinking analysis, resulting in a native talent for understanding others' points of view and objectively arriving at compromise and resolution. They tend to be deep thinkers and circumspect; they aren't given to shouting their views from the rooftops. While Earth/Metals may be reluctant to embrace change, their thoughtfulness and knack for critical thought make them receptive to a well-developed argument for change. Earth/Metal types will be more structured in their endeavors. If gardening is the hobby, the garden will be organized according to colors, height, or category. They are eager to share the fruits of their work with those around them. Their love of the finer things in life is a reflection of the Metal influence.

One of my clients epitomizes the Earth/Metal type. She is Mother Earth to every employee in our salon and spa, yet she is extremely punctual for her appointments and expects every technician to be the same. She often volunteers to assist in our business during the busy holiday seasons and is quick to organize every detail of the gift certificate center. Every package that leaves the area must have a flower or holiday berry; every detail matches from the color of the ribbon to the color of the ink on the certificates. Her genuine concern for our company, clients, employees, and those around her brings serenity to our environment whenever she is present. Her calendar is planned a year in advance as she is busy with international travel as well as travel throughout the United States. She is meticulous in planning and organization down to the smallest detail, which is a Metal element trait. Her love of the arts, fine wine, beautiful objects, museums, and designer clothing also reflects her Metal element while her warmth and generosity are Earth traits. She exemplifies a balanced Earth/Metal type which is a very productive combination.

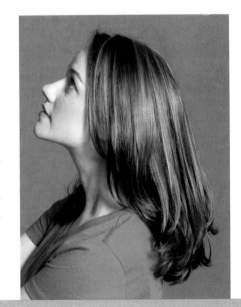

Harmonize Earth/Metal 2

If you measure Yin Extreme or 2 on the Element Barometer, you will need to add Fire. Your Earth element needs the added spark from Fire in order to become balanced. It is the extra boost of Fire that releases the Earth that needs encouragement. Be careful when adding Fire as your Earth/Metal type will need a gradual introduction to Fire instead of a Fire makeover.

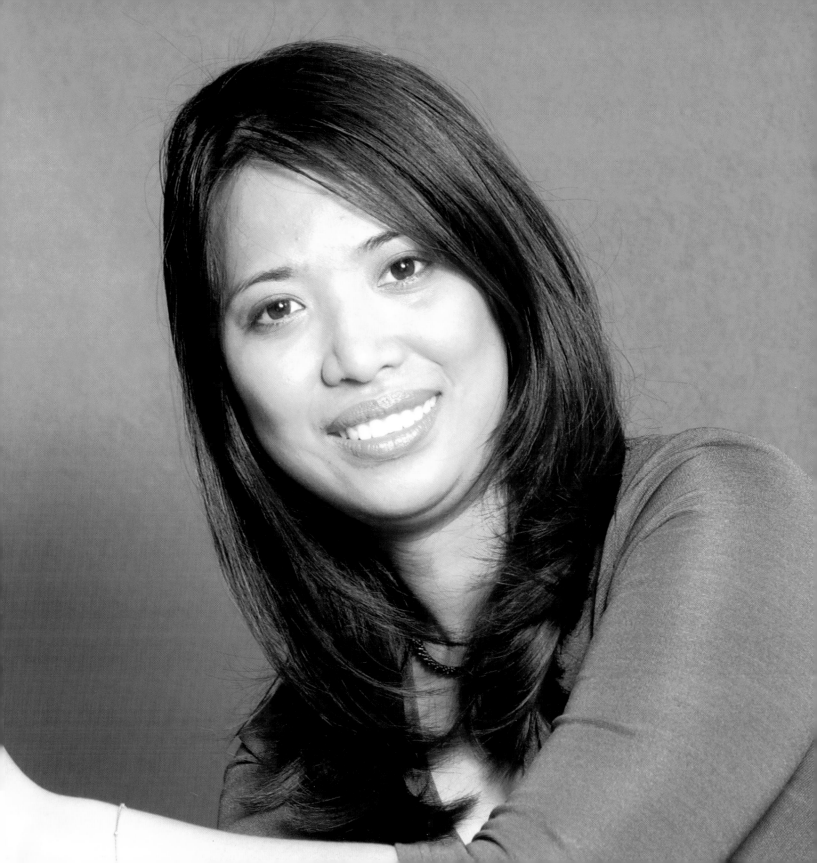

Haircut to Harmonize Earth/Metal 2

Harmonize with Fire to add texture in an orderly pattern. Earth haircuts are natural with clean lines while Metal haircuts are controlled with not a hair out of place. Fire haircuts are expressive with texture or disconnected and uneven pieces creating the style. You want to get a modified Fire haircut that creates texture without chaos. Refer to Chapter 11: Hairstyling for Your Body Type, Face Shape, and Facial Features for the best cuts.

Hair color to Harmonize Earth/Metal 2

Harmonize with Fire by creating Fire highlights. Refer to Chapter 11: Hairstyling for Your Body Type, Face Shape, and Facial Features for proper placement and application. I recommend a random pattern of back-to-back slices for highlights. Select hair color from Chapter 12: Skin Tone and Hair Color. It is vital that you know your skin tone when selecting your hair colors. With the Fire element, your only limitation in selecting a hair color is your skin tone. If you have a warm skin tone, you will want to select hair colors that are warm. You can wear any hair color as long as it is a warm tone. You have a wide array of colors available, but I recommend honoring your Earth/Metal element when making a color selection by not going too far away from your natural range.

Enhance Earth/Metal 4

If you measure Yin Moderate or 4 on the Element Barometer, you need to enhance your element by adding more Earth. You state that you are an Earth element, but your look may not project Earth element techniques or colors. Your Earth element may be depleted and in need of pampering or having someone do something for you. If so, don't hesitate to accept someone's offer to massage your back or rub your feet. It is just as important to learn how to receive as to give.

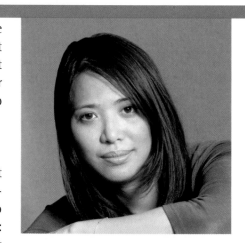

Haircut to Enhance Earth/Metal 4

Enhance with Earth for a soft, simple, and semi-classic look. You don't want to select a style that is too natural as you also have the Metal element influence to consider. Instead of wearing your hair all one length, you may want to select a style that has some light texture for movement. Refer to Chapter 11: Hairstyling for Your Body Type, Face Shape, and Facial Features for the best haircut. Remember that Earth style does not mean a dowdy look or like someone who just runs a comb through her hair and is finished for the day. You will want softer lines around your face for an Earth haircut than if you were to select one with Metal influence.

Hair color to Enhance Earth/Metal 4

Enhance with Earth highlighting techniques and refer to Chapter 11: Hair-styling for Your Body Type, Face Shape, and Facial Features for the proper placement and application techniques. With Earth highlighting techniques, you use four to six pieces per pickup. With Metal highlighting techniques, you use seven to nine pieces per pickup. I would recommend using six to seven pieces per pickup for a refined, precise look. Refer to Chapter 12: Skin Tone and Hair Color for your color selection. If you are a natural level six, you may select colors from level four or five, or seven or eight. You are the one to decide if you want to go a shade lighter or darker. Make certain that you know your skin tone as it may vary with the seasons depending on the amount of time you spend in the sun.

Harmonize Earth/Metal 6

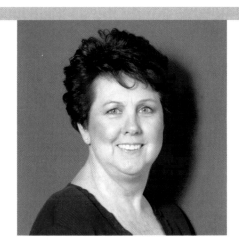

If you measure Yang Moderate or 6 on the Element Barometer, you need to add Metal for a classic style in your cut or color. The Metal element assists the Earth/Metal type in making decisions quickly and deliberately. Metal element also helps to stabilize Earth. As a Yang Moderate, you have too much Earth and need to decrease or lessen the Earth element's influence by adding Metal. Add a Metal element cut, color, or makeup to sharpen your look and give a more classic appearance. Look at your environment and your life. Is your desk, room, car, or closet organized or full of clutter? To gain more control of your life, spend time organizing and freeing your living space of unwanted items. Discarding items that you no longer wear or use will enable you to become more productive. When using a Metal element haircut, color, or makeup, you must feel comfortable with the addition of a more precise look. You make the decision on how much Metal to add to your look.

Haircut to Harmonize Earth/Metal 6

Harmonize with Metal by selecting a classic look that uses softening shears to create a soft texture. Make certain that your haircut does not have the sharp lines or edges of a classic Metal cut. You are striving for a Metal adaptation for your Earth element. Refer to Chapter 11: Hairstyling for Your Body Type, Face Shape, and Facial Features for the best cut for you.

Hair color to Harmonize Earth/Metal 6

Harmonize with Metal highlighting techniques that require refined back-to-back slices. Refer to Chapter 12: Skin Tone and Hair Color for your color selection.

Please make certain that you check the section on skin tone definitions before turning to the Metal colors. If you are a natural level five, you may select colors from levels two through four or six through nine. The Metal element has a wide range of colors for selection. It is vital that you look at the different levels and tones before making a selection. Unless you select a semi-permanent color which will wash out gradually in three to four weeks, you will have the color you select for six to eight weeks. Look at Chapter 11: Hairstyling for Your Body Type, Face Shape, and Facial Features for highlighting techniques and application.

Balance Earth/Metal 8

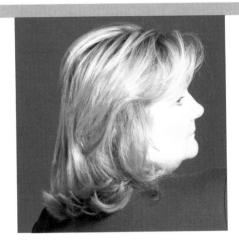

If you measure Yang Extreme or 8 on the Element Barometer, you are displaying too much Earth and need to add Wood for balance, but you must be cautious about how much of the Wood element you add. Balance is the key component in deciding how much Wood to add. I recommend adding activities and hobbies that give you the opportunity to be with others in a social setting. When you have too much Earth and Metal, you become rigid and unyielding as you tend to turn inward. The Wood element is more social and outgoing and provides an excellent way for you to seek balance on your own terms.

Haircut to Balance Earth/Metal 8

Balance with Wood by selecting a cut that adds texture for a tousled look. You want to select an expressive cut that has style without restrictions. Wood cuts are designed to have movement. Refer to Chapter 11: Hairstyling for Your Body Type, Face Shape, and Facial Features for the best cut. A Wood cut will have more freedom and texture that an Earth or Metal haircut.

Hair color to Balance Earth/Metal 8

Balance by using the Wood techniques as described in Chapter 12: Skin Tone and Hair Color and refer to the selection of colors for your natural level. If you are a natural level eight, you may select colors from levels six or seven, or nine through eleven. It is vital that you are accurate in determining your skin tone as your skin tone may vary according to the amount of time spent in the sun. Wood highlighting techniques are sporty and will allow for more variance of color throughout your hair. I recommend using two to three different colors for your hair to add depth.

Earth/Water

You've heard that still waters run deep; predictably, Earth/Water people tend to suppress their heartfelt feelings and desires. These types are more apt to think and meditate before expressing their emotions or acting upon their feelings. The more emotional of the Earth combinations, these people tend to have abundant curiosities that can focus on world issues or on the trials and tribulations of their inner circle. Earth/Water people would be the ones who not only watch the news and read the media about current issues but who also research the background that created the issue. They seek knowledge in order to help make the world, their country, and their community a better place to live. It is vital that these types are aware of their outside pressures as well as the ones they create.

Earth/Water types crave protection and security, as they're wired to protect and nurture others. It is not unusual for these types to seek refuge in nature by going away to a mountain cabin with nothing but their books for company and a journal to record their thoughts. They can quote the works of philosophers who made an impression on their lives and their values. They give of their time and energy so freely that it is in books, education, and nature that they find their solitude and replenish their souls. If they fail to take time for themselves away from outside influences, it may affect their health. They may be torn between emotional curiosity and the desire to remain unchanged and safe.

Earth/Water types have the ability to make a difference in the lives of those they touch. When they are in balance, they have the compassion and the ability to think positively that can turn around others who seem to wander aimlessly. Their demeanor is calming to those seeking an anchor in their lives. If they are not in balance, they find it difficult to get along with anyone and become suspicious of the motives of others. These types must make time in their daily lives for a quiet spot to drink a cup of tea and read or reflect on the day. For the Earth/Water types to function at their highest potential they have to take some time with no interruptions.

Harmonize Earth/Water 2

If you measure Yin Extreme or 2 on the Element Barometer, you need to add Fire to create more Earth and to increase its intensity. I recommend adding Fire gradually to change your appearance. I begin with a Fire haircut, color, or highlights. Also, you may add Fire by finding a way to release your artistic talents. It may be in your garden, painting your home, clothing or your accessories.

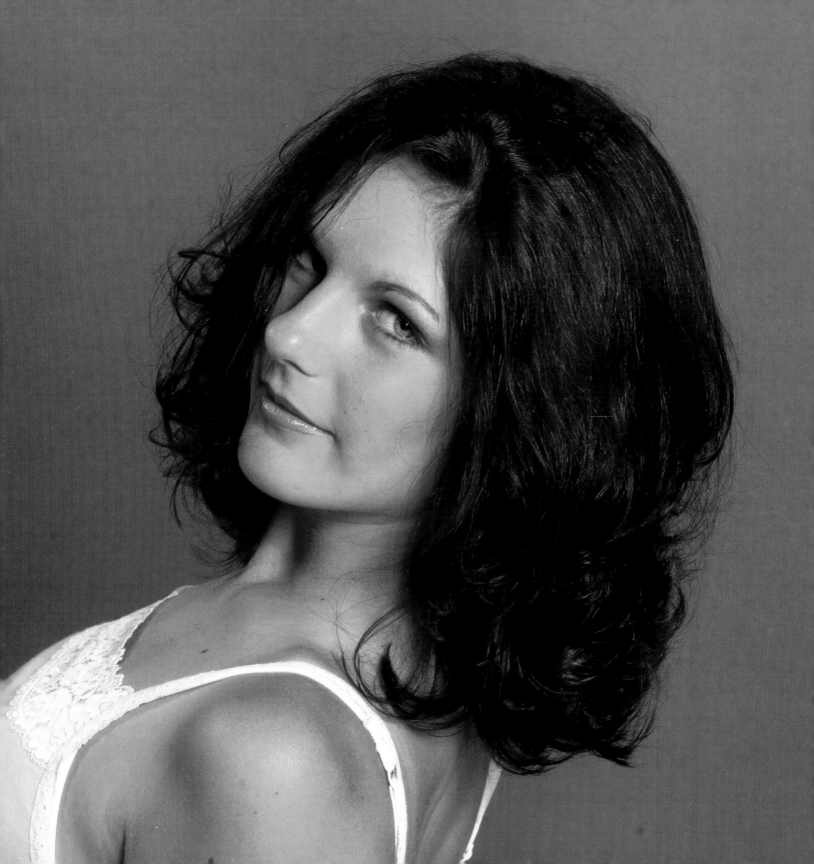

Haircut to Harmonize Earth/Water 2

Harmonize with Fire to create an attitude by using uneven or disconnected pieces in a long cut or choppy pieces in a short cut. Refer to Chapter 11: Hairstyling for Your Body Type, Face Shape, and Facial Features for the best cut for you. If you prefer a more subtle Fire haircut, you may want to try using a petal cutting technique that creates movement and texture without a sharp edge.

Hair color to Harmonize Earth/Water 2

Harmonize with Fire by selecting a deeper or brighter color depending on the season and your skin tone. Refer to Chapter 12: Skin Tone and Hair Color for the color selection. Your only limitation in selecting a color is your skin tone. With the Fire element, you can choose any color. From Chapter 11: Hairstyling for Your Body Type, Face Shape, and Facial Features, select the highlighting techniques and placement of the highlights. I recommend using slicing techniques according to your facial shape.

Enhance Earth/Water 4

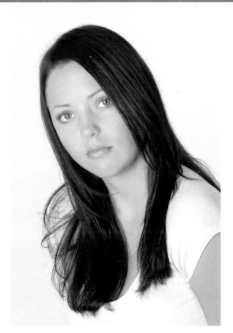

If you measure Yin Moderate or 4 on the Element Barometer, you will want to add Earth for enrichment. Earth types are gentle, supportive, and caring for the world around them. You can become so much a part of the lives of others that you have a difficult time honoring who you are. It is important for you to exercise and find time to take care of your health. Often, you will take care of others to the detriment of your appearance, your immediate family, health, and diet. You have always spent your time caring for others and thought or were taught that it is selfish to think about yourself. Spend at least fifteen minutes every morning and evening for you—it may be the first thing in the morning or the last thing at night. You may want to read, meditate, write, or listen to music. It is your time.

Haircut to Enhance Earth/Water 4

Enhance with Earth by creating a one-length haircut for longer hair. If you desire a short hair, cut the hair close to the head following its natural shape. Refer to Chapter 11: Hairstyling for Your Body Type, Face Shape, and Facial Features for the best cut. Your goal is to create a hairstyle that does not detract from who you are, but rather one that enhances your natural beauty.

Hair color to Enhance Earth/Water 4

Enhance with Earth by referring to Chapter 12: Skin Tone and Hair Color for your color selection. If you are a natural level six, you may select colors from levels four or five, or seven or eight depending on your skin tone. Coloring techniques and placement are found in Chapter 11: Hairstyling for Your Body Type, Face Shape, and Facial Features. You may select Water or Earth highlighting techniques. When using Water highlighting techniques, you may choose to use one to three colors to create depth. Make certain the colors are from the same family of colors.

Harmonize Earth/Water 6

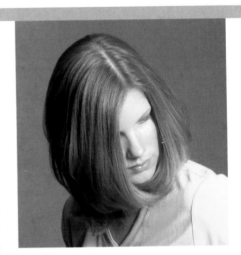

If you measure Yang Moderate or 6 on the Element Barometer, you need to add Metal for balance. Your Earth element needs structure and organization in order to function at its highest potential. When the Earth element becomes too involved with others and stuck in the present, it needs schedules and procedures to stabilize it. I recommend adding Metal to your lifestyle, clothing, and hobbies as well as to your haircut, color, and makeup. It is up to you how much Metal you add. You must feel comfortable and embrace the changes in your life in order for them to be positive. For this reason I recommend your take it one step at a time.

Haircut to Harmonize Earth/Water 6

Harmonize with Metal by selecting a sleek sophisticated style that uses softening shears for a tapered line instead of a well-defined or severe line. Refer to Chapter 11: Hairstyling for Your Body Type, Face Shape, and Facial Features for the best cut for you. A Metal haircut will be more structured than an Earth cut—go with as much structure as you're comfortable with.

Hair color to Harmonize Earth/Water 6

Harmonize with Metal by referring to Chapter 12: Skin Tone and Hair Color for your color selection. If you are a natural level six, you may select colors from levels three through five or seven through ten. By looking at Chapter 11: Hairstyling for Your Body Type, Face Shape, and Facial Features you will find highlighting techniques and placement. I recommend using one eighth slices for the highlighting utilizing from two to three colors for depth.

Balance Earth/Water 8

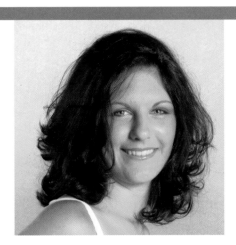

If you measure Yang Extreme or 8 on the Element Barometer, you need to balance with Wood element in your look and lifestyle. A Yang Extreme indicates your Chi is blocked and your warm gentle demeanor is not coming through. Wood element types are very active and always on the go. You need to become more involved with others and seek activities that include more social contact. I recommend that you set your personal and professional goals and create a plan on when and how you will achieve them. Wood element types are great leaders and more than willing to deliver a speech at a moment's notice. Wood will definitely bring energy to Earth/Water if you accept it willingly.

Haircut to Balance Earth/Water 8

Balance with Wood by adding texture for movement and volume. Wood types seek a professional look that suggests movement. With longer hairstyles, create long rounded layers that frame the face. Refer to Chapter 11: Hairstyling for Your Body Type, Face Shape, and Facial Features for the correct length and style for you. Short hairstyles will have the most texture of any of the element cuts.

Hair color to Balance Earth/Water 8

Balance with Wood by using Wood highlighting techniques from Chapter 12: Skin Tone and Hair Color. This chapter will also give you your color selection. With the Wood element, you can select two to three colors for your highlighting. If you are a natural level four, you may select colors from levels two or three, or five through seven. The Wood element is a fun, active element so feel free to select colors and techniques that denote this freedom while still maintaining a professional look if you desire.

Earth/Wood

Earth/Wood types are often marked by the duality of their impulse for optimism and their tendency to cling to safe, known routines. The contradiction of these traits may make it easier for them to cope with change when surrounded by the security and safety of a familiar group. Earth/Wood types are nurturing with their family, friends, and coworkers. Their concern for the well-being of those around them usually dominates their actions. On the other hand, they can be fiercely competitive in seeking to achieve their goals. They will compete against themselves and push to be better and better. They are not the ones to rest on last year's laurels. As leaders, they become creative in designing contests for their coworkers to increase productivity. The contests as well as the prizes are fun and create good will among those involved.

Since Earth people thrive in familiar surroundings and environment, they are more receptive to change with a Wood influence. Wood influences welcome change and the opportunity to travel and seek new adventurers. One of our salon managers is an Earth/Wood type. She is very soft-spoken and evokes warmth whenever she enters a room. Her confident demeanor and genuine concern for others creates a welcoming environment for our employees and clients. Her staff loves the challenge of creating new treatments and packages and are always at the top in any contest. This Earth/Wood type is enthusiastic about new ideas and is quick to implement them with her staff.

Harmonize Earth/Wood 2

If you measure Yin Extreme or 2 on the Element Barometer, add Fire element to create new energy. You want to add more expression to your style whether it is in clothing, accessories, haircut or color, or makeup. Don't be afraid to experiment with bold colors and daring new looks. Find an artistic release in dancing, painting, sculpting, singing, playing an instrument, or any other activity that requires your creativity. You will never know how great you can be if you don't step outside of the box and take a chance.

Haircut to Harmonize Earth/Wood 2

Harmonize with Fire by adding texture while striving for an edgier cut. If you have long hair, add texture to the top with longer bangs brushed to the side. You want movement throughout the hair—a wild look that promises excitement. For short hair, select a disconnected look that accentuates your eyes or frames your face. Have fun with styling products to create different looks. Refer

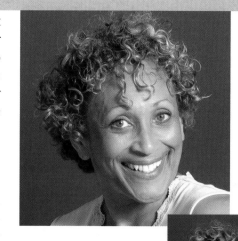

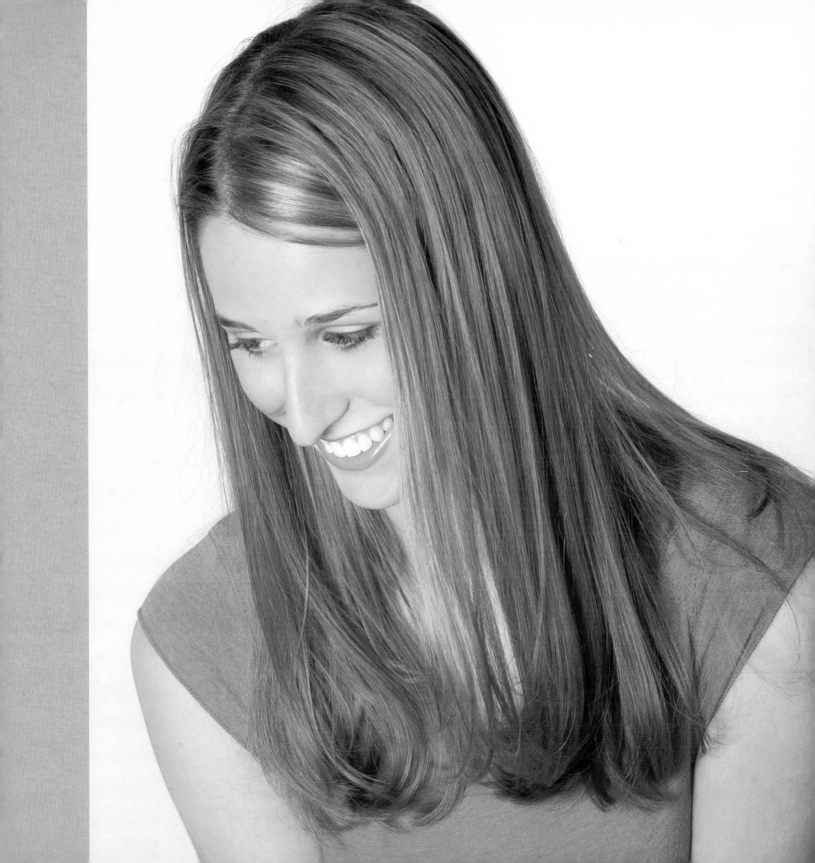

to Chapter 11: Hairstyling for Your Body Type, Face Shape, and Facial Features for the cuts that will look great on you.

Hair color to Harmonize Earth/Wood 2

Harmonize with Fire by selecting bold colors from Chapter 12: Skin Tone and Hair Color. Your skin tone and your desire to have a makeover are your only limitations on color. Refer to Chapter 11: Hairstyling for Your Body Type, Face Shape, and Facial Features for highlighting techniques and placement. 1 recommend starting with a few Fire highlighting techniques around your face if your face shape allows it. 1 would suggest that you not have a Fire color and full Fire highlights unless you are completely sure you are ready for it.

Enhance Earth/Wood 4

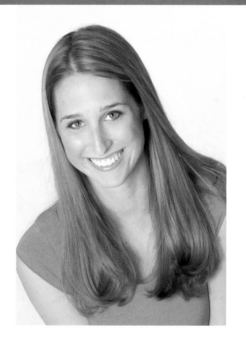

If you measure Yin Moderate or 4 on the Element Barometer, you will need to add Earth to enhance or bring out more of the Earth element. You may appear reserved and shy at first meeting and may be reluctant to share your ideas unless you are confident they'll be met with a warm reception. With the addition of more enrichment, or more Earth, you are able to replenish yourself. Take time to pamper yourself. Prepare your favorite meal for a change or select the movie you want to see. Earth types usually defer to others when preparing meals or selecting any type of entertainment. If you don't make the time to take care of you, it will affect your mental, emotional, and physical health.

Haircut to Enhance Earth/Wood 4

Enhance with Earth by adding more texture for a dancing movement. You are looking for slight natural movement. Refer to Chapter 11: Hairstyling for Your Body Type, Face Shape, and Facial Features for the best length and cuts. If your hair is curly, you can wear it any length according to your facial shape. 1 recommend cutting into the curl to allow it to have more spring.

Hair color to Enhance Earth/Wood 4

Enhance with Earth by selecting colors from Chapter 12: Skin Tone and Hair Color. If you are a natural level four, you may select colors and tones from level two or three, or five or six. You may want to change your colors with the seasons—level two or three for the fall and winter. This will give you a deeper and darker color. For highlighting techniques refer to Chapter 11: Hairstyling for Your Body Type, Face Shape, and Facial Features for placement application.

Harmonize Earth/Wood 6

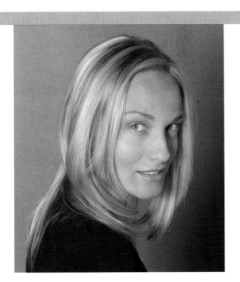

If you measure Yang Moderate or 6 the Element Barometer, introduce Metal to bring order and discipline to Earth/Wood types. Metal types enjoy working within guidelines and knowing their boundaries. In order for the Earth/Wood type to meet deadlines, it is crucial to add Metal which helps to solidify ideas and bring them to fruition. Making lists and time lines helps to keep an Earth/Wood type on schedule. If not, they have a hard time saying no when others want their time and energy. Follow-through is difficult for Earth/Wood types without the addition of Metal. The amount of Metal or structure that is needed is an individual matter and can change with experiences, so go with what feels right for you.

Haircut to Harmonize Earth/Wood 6

Harmonize with Metal for a softened classy look; strive for a more feminine style. Select the classic Metal cut, but you want a softer line, not so sharp and defined. The key to a Metal cut is perfection without any hair out of place. It never looks windblown on purpose. Refer to Chapter 11: Hairstyling for Your Body Type, Face Shape, and Facial Features for the best way to achieve this cut.

Hair color to Harmonize Earth/Wood 6

Harmonize with Metal by referring to Chapter 12: Skin Tone and Hair Color for the color selection. Make certain that you know your skin tone as the colors will vary according to skin tone. If you have a warm Milky skin tone, you will have different color selections available than a cool Porcelain skin tone. Your skin tone may change depending on the amount of time you spend in the sun. If you are a natural level six, you may select colors from levels three through five or seven through ten. Turn to Chapter 11: Hairstyling for Your Body Type, Face Shape, and Facial Features for highlighting placement and techniques.

Balance Earth/Wood 8

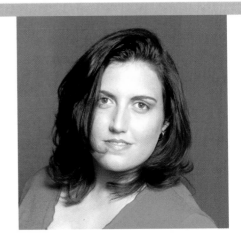

If you measure Yang Extreme or 8 on the Element Barometer, use the Wood element to balance. Wood element types are more open and outgoing than Earth types. By adding hobbies and outdoor activities that are in a social setting you will become more involved with others and not so reluctant to learn new ideas and try new things. The addition of Wood in your looks and your lifestyle will add a new dimension and permit you to become more free and receptive to fresh new ideas and fashion. This is the perfect opportunity for you to make a change in one or all aspects of your appearance.

Haircut to Balance Earth/Wood 8

Balance with Wood in your cut by rounding layers for movement. You want to create movement within the haircut. Cut into the hair for texture and to create volume. Refer to Chapter 11: Hairstyling for Your Body Type, Face Shape, and Facial Features for the best cut and length.

Hair color to Balance Earth/Wood 8

Balance with Wood by referring to Chapter 12: Skin Tone and Hair Color for color selection. If you are a natural level seven, you may select colors from levels five or six, or eight through ten. Look in Chapter 11: Hairstyling for Your Body Type, Face Shape, and Facial Features for highlighting placement and application. You can be more expressive with your Wood techniques since your lifestyle element is also Wood. Remember to check your skin tone with the change of the seasons as your skin tone will change with sun exposure.

8 Metal Element

Metal types like the facts—just the facts. Don't bother them with descriptive language and explanations. Flowery poetry filled with imagery and beautiful language does not interest Metal types. Although Metal types love to ask questions, they are not receptive to answering what they consider frivolous questions. Do not involve them in idle chitchat. Metal types enjoy crossword puzzles, chess, and any other activity that involves intellectual acuity. They are highly disciplined and detail-oriented which can be an asset or liability depending on the level of their obsession. People with too much Metal often don't focus on current events or family; they are absorbed with their projects and are not easily distracted by others.

If you need a project completed on time and accurately, a Metal type will answer the call. They can focus their attention and complete any task. People who are Metal are usually very neat and dislike clutter. Their closets, dressers, desks, and cars are usually organized, clean, and clutter-free. It is rare for Metal types to be able to multitask, as they dedicate their efforts and attention to their current project.

An example of the Metal type is a gentleman who is a close friend of mine. He is always impeccably dressed and prefers traditional classic fashion. His obsession about the smallest detail will extend any project beyond the amount of time that one would expect. He becomes so absorbed in the task—whether it is his work, gardening, remodeling the home, or working a crossword puzzle—that he forgets the time. His opinions are very conservative and based on a solid foundation according to his research. Change is very hard for him to accept, especially when deviating from a planned schedule. If he is surrounded with clutter, he becomes distracted and is unable to perform to his satisfaction. In fact, he may become distracted when cleaning his desk and spend hours reading old files and articles. In his profession as a medical sales representative, his thirst for knowledge about the products was not limited to what was necessary to communicate to the physician, but extended into the research of the product and in-depth knowledge of the ingredients. It is extremely difficult for him to relax, and I have never seen him in sloppy attire or even looking casual. His dominant element of Metal is reflected in every aspect of his life.

Metal types are usually experts on anything that interests them. If they become interested in fine wines, they will know the year, type, and best brand of wine available.

They rarely take the advice of others and prefer to heed their own counsel. Pride and confidence are evident in a balanced Metal type. They are not tolerant of anyone who fails to live up to their standards and can become inflexible in their demands.

I value our Metal employees, as they bring structure to the creative world of beauty. While most people would think that hair designers are more the Fire types, the Metal designers are the ones who run on time, and their clients usually do the same. Their stations are organized with the drawers neatly arranged. They never think of using a tube of color without replacing the cap and putting the tube back into its proper place. They never borrow anyone else's tools without asking first and always return them immediately after using. Their method of cutting is precise and their hair colors are always consistent. Whenever they are introduced to a new technique or style, they study and practice it until they have learned it to their satisfaction before they will perform it on a client. In our corporate office, our payroll and accounting departments are staffed with Metal types as there is no room for errors on employee paychecks or in accounting.

When Metal types select a sport or physical activity, they become totally dedicated to reaching their highest potential. They have the discipline and drive to adhere to a strict schedule and diet or whatever is required for them to excel. In order for the Metal types to stay balanced, they need to seek social activities where they have the opportunity to unwind and relax. Improvisation, impromptu, or extemporaneous behavior is totally out of character for a Metal type. If they do something that seems spur-of-the moment, it probably has been planned in secret. They strive for perfection and it is a lofty goal.

Within each element, Yin and Yang energies exist. On the Element Barometer, I have listed characteristics that will assist you in knowing whether you need to enhance, harmonize, or balance the element. If the Metal element is hidden or Yin Extreme 2, you need to add the Earth element for a softer, more natural look. When the Yin is Moderate 4, you need to enhance the Metal. If the Yang is Moderate 6, you need to add Water, slowing down the Metal. When the Metal element is too extreme—Yang 8—I recommend using Fire to balance or control the Metal. The degree of Metal that we express can be compared to the different types of Metal we use. Carbon iron, used in cutting tools and other items where strength is required, is extremely hard to bend. That would be similar to a Yang Extreme 8 on the Element Barometer. A Yang Moderate Metal 6 is similar to steel that is used in cookware and heavy machinery; it is more malleable than iron. A Yin Moderate Metal 4 is much like the aluminum that is used for the framework of buildings and transportation vehicles. A Yin Extreme Metal 2 is more malleable, like the gold used to make our jewelry.

Using Feng Shui principles designed to bring balance or create a flow of good Chi, I take into consideration not only your haircut, hair color, makeup, body type, and face shape but also your hobbies, your lifestyle, your exercise patterns, meditation, clothing, and accessories. All of these things affect you and the image you portray. When I prescribe the look that will best reflect how you perceive yourself, I also make recommendations to other factors that influence your life. Some of the changes or recommendations will be evident almost immediately such as haircut, hair color, and makeup. The other changes will involve more of your participation and will evolve, as you are the one in charge of implementing that part of your life. The amount of change will depend upon your dedication.

Makeup for the Metal element

You use more classic colors as well as techniques. The only restriction is your skin tone. Makeup is a way to create a new look that can change with your moods. I recommend that you follow your instinct when selecting colors and techniques. Metal makeup is referred to as pretty, flawless, and classic. Your element strives for perfection in your appearance.

Porcelain

Use mauve, pink, lavender, light blue, or blue gray eye shadow with gray blue eyeliner. Lip colors should be red to nude.

Milky

Use brown liner with ivory to peach shadows on eyelids. Lips should be more peach to nude.

Honey

Try brown liner with brown eye shadow. You can add ivory or cream to lids. Go rust to brown to nude on your lips, depending on the season.

Olive

Apply russet red brown or mauve shadow and berry, cinnamon, or deep red lip color.

Ebony

Russet red-brown shadow will work well on eyes, with lips brown-red.

Ruby

Use a brown liner for smoky eyes and color lips brown or berry.

Metal/Fire

Metal/Fire types will volunteer for any new project and complete it. They are ready to assist when asked. If you need someone to lift your spirits, call your Metal/Fire friend. They do not, however, know how to balance their personal, professional, and social responsibilities, and are likely to burn out rather than ask for help.

Metal/Fire types enjoy being asked for their opinions and will readily express them. They rarely volunteer their opinions unless it is with their close circle of friends or coworkers. If Metal/Fire types are in balance, they can be great at business, combining discipline with creativity and passion.

One of my friends and clients is a Metal/Fire type. He is focused at work and thrives on growing his business. He owns an organic produce company that ships internationally. His standard for producing an organic product that has the nutrients needed for a healthy diet has made him a pioneer and leader in the industry. He has his stamp on all aspects of his business, from marketing, planting, and harvesting to transporting the produce to its final destination. After harvest or a long day at work, he is ready to play. He plays just as hard as he works and loves showering his friends with gifts. Whether it is gathering friends at his home for a pool party or flying them in his airplane or bringing them to opening night at the theater, he loves being surrounded by laughter and music. He could have excelled at a career in singing, dancing, or any field in the entertainment industry; however, his family business needed a strong leader and he rose to the occasion.

Harmonize Metal/Fire 2

If you measure Yin Extreme or 2 on the Element Barometer, you need to feed the Metal by adding Earth. You need to add Earth to boost the Metal to make it stronger. Earth will give it a strong foundation of values and an uncomplicated style. A Metal type may become too intense, withdrawn, and indecisive when it needs replenishing. By adding Earth to Metal, you increase the strength of the Metal. Think about how you spend your leisure time. I recommend that you volunteer your time for a charity or plant a garden of vegetables or flowers to share with your friends. The goal of Feng Shui is to bring you into balance in all aspects of your life.

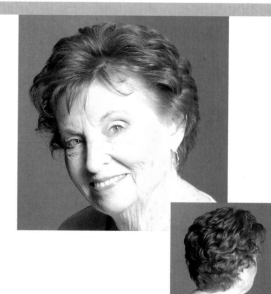

Haircut to Harmonize Metal/Fire 2
Harmonize with Earth by seeking a classic cut with softened lines. Seek a clean line with your haircut that does not require a lot of time to style. If your hair

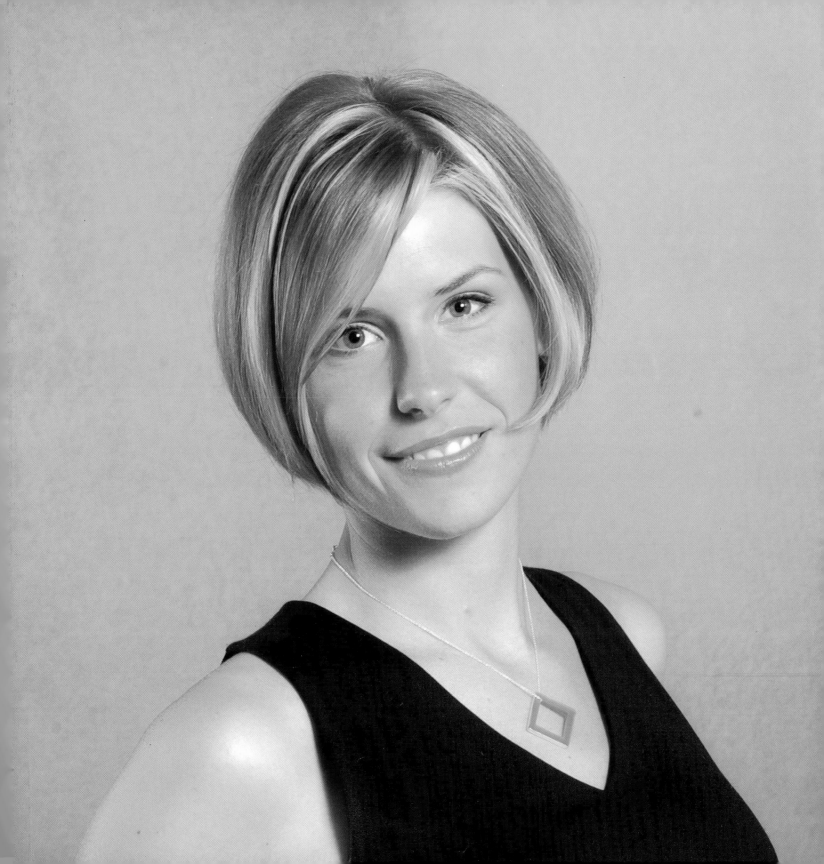

is curly, let it hang naturally. Cut into the ends for movement and add texture for volume. Refer to Chapter 11: Hairstyling for Your Body Type, Face Shape, and Facial Features for the best length, cut, and cutting techniques. The key component to the look will be natural or soft movement in the style.

Hair color to Harmonize Metal/Fire 2

Harmonize with Earth by following the color selections in Chapter 12: Skin Tone and Hair Color. Make the colors close to your natural level. If you are a natural level five, you may select colors from level three or four, or six or seven. Refer to Chapter 11: Hairstyling for Your Body Type, Face Shape, and Facial Features for highlighting techniques and placement. With highlighting, you may use two to three colors within the same color family. Earth highlighting techniques use four to six pieces per pickup for a natural effect.

Enhance Metal/Fire 4

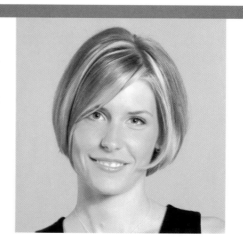

If you measure Yin Moderate or 4 on the Element Barometer, you need to add more Metal or structure in your life and style. I recommend adding a Metal haircut and color in order to enhance your predominant element. Honor your secondary element by deciding how much structure you feel comfortable with. You can enhance your lifestyle by listening to classical music, visiting an art gallery, or learning a new skill that requires mental acuity.

Haircut to Enhance Metal/Fire 4

Enhance with Metal by selecting a style with fine detailing and classic lines with a shattered edge. Refer to Chapter 11: Hairstyling for Your Body Type, Face Shape, and Facial Features for the best haircut. If you have curly hair, I recommend a graduated bob depending on your face shape. Cut into the crown for volume and into the rest of your hair if it is heavy with curls. Strive for a soft, classic look.

Hair color to Enhance Metal/Fire 4

Colors should be classic and enhance your beauty. Refer to Chapter 12: Skin Tone and Hair Color for the wide array of colors available to you. If you are a natural level six, you may select from levels three though five or seven through ten. For highlighting, refer to Chapter 11: Hairstyling for Your Body Type, Face Shape, and Facial Features. You want precise highlights for a sun-kissed look to the style.

Harmonize Metal/Fire 6

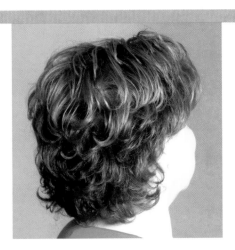

If you measure Yang Moderate or 6 on the Element Barometer, you will need to introduce the Water element for some energy and chic to the cuts and color. Add some Water to your life by perusing the shelves at the local bookstore for the latest book on the future or on meditation. Water helps to slow down the pace of Metal/Fire types by causing them to reflect before acting. Water types are more open to change and to new ideas. Water fashions add an extra kick or flair that may be missing from Metal types. The Water element is perfect to harmonize Metal/Fire.

Haircut to Harmonize Metal/Fire 6

Harmonize with Water by selecting a sassy, mischievous style which allows texture to create a sensual look. This will be a very new look for a Metal/Fire type—although the Fire influence is definitely game for this type of change. Refer to Chapter 11: Hairstyling for Your Body Type, Face Shape, and Facial Features for the best haircut.

Hair color to Harmonize Metal/Fire 6

Harmonize with Water colors by turning to Chapter 12: Skin Tone and Hair Color for your color selection. If you are a natural level seven, you may select colors from levels three through six or eight through eleven. Chapter 11: Hairstyling for Your Body Type, Face Shape, and Facial Features contains highlighting techniques and placement. I recommend using the Monet technique as it uses three colors from the same family for a soft look.

Balance Metal/Fire 8

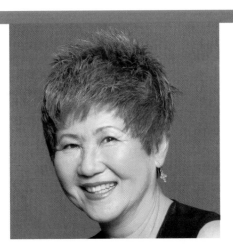

If you measure Yang Extreme or 8 on the Element Barometer, add Fire to melt or make the Metal more pliable. You want to balance the Metal/Fire element. If Metal is Yang Extreme, it means that you have become rigid and opinionated. If you don't introduce fun into your life, you run the risk of damaging your health. Fire element is about enjoying the moment with a lot of zest. Learn a new dance, sing in your shower, paint your room a vibrant color, and shout to the world that you are alive. You decide when and how much Fire element you want to introduce into your appearance and life. Feng Shui is all about bringing balance into your life and honoring your decisions.

Haircut to Balance Metal/Fire 8

Balance with Fire by adding texture and uneven pieces in a classic cut. Slightly shatter the lines of the style for a freer and fun style. Refer to Chapter 11: Hairstyling for Your Body Type, Face Shape, and Facial Features for the best hair cut and length. If you have curly hair, the cut will depend upon how tight your curls are. You may want to straighten or soften the curl by cutting into the hair. Select the technique for finding the root jump. This technique allows the curls to move within a style. Strive for a creative cut that suits your element.

Hair color to Balance Metal/Fire 8

Balance with Fire highlights as recommended in Chapter 11: Hairstyling for Your Body Type, Face Shape, and Facial Features. Be as bold as you dare when selecting Fire techniques. Refer to Chapter 12: Skin Tone and Hair Color for your color selection. With the Fire element, you may select any color as long as it matches your skin tone.

Metal/Earth

Metal/Earth types have a difficult time making decisions. They spend endless hours discussing and researching the possibilities rather than taking action. They have a great deal of patience whenever they get stuck while working on a task. This Metal/Earth combination will assist others when asked for guidance. They make great friends, as they are concerned about your needs and will listen when you talk—really listen, looking you in the eye. They can repeat what you have said as they have great capacity to focus. If you need help, they are ready for action. They thrive on the innocence of children and take great joy in their achievements. Rather than painting a picture, they enjoy spending hours in a museum or art gallery observing and appreciating the exhibits. They can accept new information but they prefer routines. When these types are balanced, it can be the best of both worlds: discipline and focus with caring and nurturing traits.

Our corporation is fortunate to have a Metal/Earth type as the senior bookkeeper. She is totally focused on entering data and balancing our accounts. Her office is totally organized even though it is crowded with filing cabinets and records. She is cautious about finances and doesn't hesitate to make everyone aware of the bottom line whenever a new project is introduced at a meeting. On the other hand, she dotes on her grandchildren and the children of the corporate employees. She will always take time to bend down to speak with them

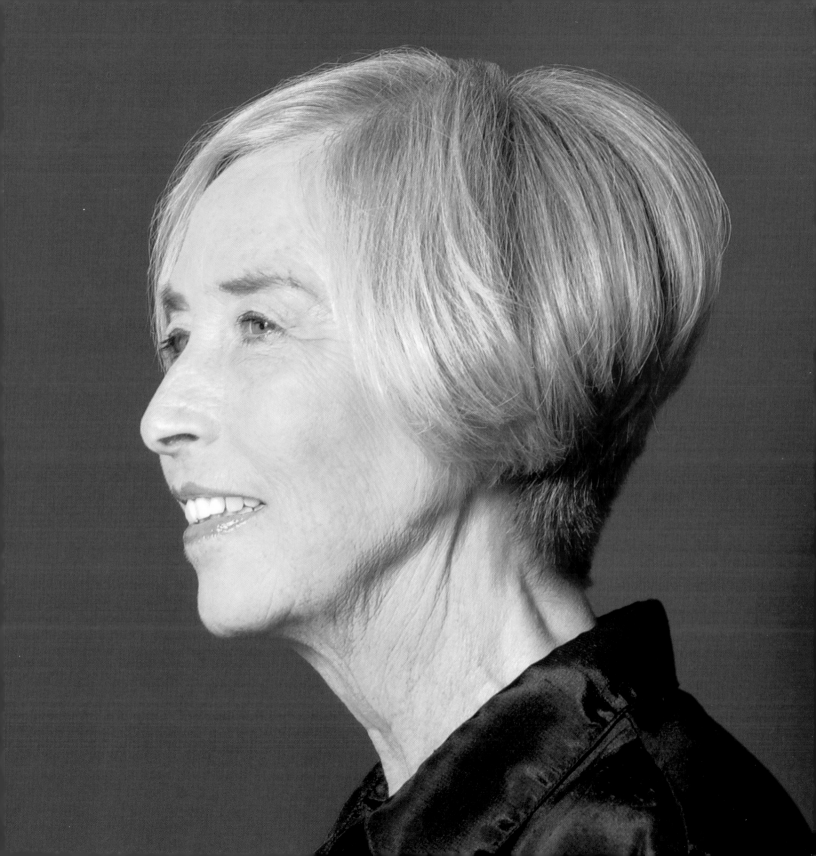

or to share her red pencil with some child who needs it to draw. She shows her concern about our company by calling in several times a day even when she is on vacation or sick. She dresses very professionally but usually wears Earth colors. Her hairstyle is very soft and cut close to her head in a structured style. She has naturally curly and wavy hair so the style is perfect for her.

Harmonize Metal/Earth 2

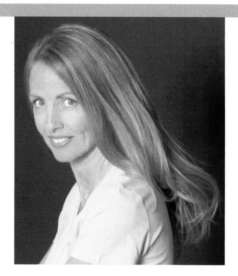

If you measure Yin Moderate or 2 on the Element Barometer, you will need to add Earth to harmonize. Earth types are calm and very stabilizing. When Metal elements become Yin Extreme, this means they are too indecisive and can become defensive and withdrawn. Introduce Earth into other aspects of your life by volunteering at a charity or scheduling a benefit for a good cause. Earth types are very family oriented and sometimes Metal types become so absorbed in their career they forget to take time for their loved ones. By adding the Earth element, it serves as a reminder to honor your loved ones and become involved in your community.

Haircut to Harmonize Metal/Earth 2

Harmonize with Earth by seeking a classic cut with softened lines. If your hair is curly, let it hang naturally and select a cut that follows your natural curl and wave. Make certain you select a style that allows a natural feel within a structured cut. Refer to Chapter 11: Hairstyling for Your Body Type, Face Shape, and Facial Features for the best haircut and length.

Hair color to Harmonize Metal/Earth 2

Harmonize with Earth by turning to Chapter 12: Skin Tone and Hair Color for Earth color selection. If you are a natural level four, you may select colors from levels two or three, or five or six. Refer to Chapter 11: Hairstyling for Your Body Type, Face Shape, and Facial Features for highlight placement, techniques, and application. It is important that you honor your predominant element of Metal by not selecting techniques that are too casual for a structured Metal/Earth type.

Enhance Metal/Earth 4

If you measure Yin Moderate or 4, you need to increase the amount of Metal in your life and appearance. Your Metal element needs to be replenished by adding more structure to your life. Set goals for your personal and professional

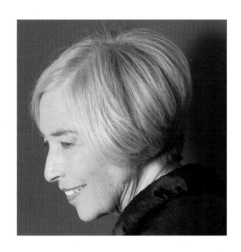

life. Devise a timeline for achieving the goals. Revisit them weekly to check on your progress. Join a gym and follow a routine at the same time each day. You need to add more discipline and a more professional look to your style. Metal element techniques for your haircut and color will be very precise and structured. You must avoid adding too much Metal as you can become too rigid and unyielding.

Haircut to Enhance Metal/Earth 4

A precision haircut with flawless structure is the ideal haircut to enhance Metal in your appearance. Refer to Chapter 11: Hairstyling for Your Body Type, Face Shape, and Facial Features for the best haircut and length. The classic bob should give you a professional appearance even if you are wearing jeans or casual attire.

Hair color to Enhance Metal/Earth 4

Enhance with tone-on-tone highlights using Metal highlighting techniques described in Chapter 12: Skin Tone and Hair Color. It is vital that you select your natural color level and that you are confident about your skin tone. If you are a natural level seven, you may select from levels four through six, or eight through eleven. Your hair color and highlights are meant to enhance your beauty and your classic style.

Harmonize Metal/Earth 6

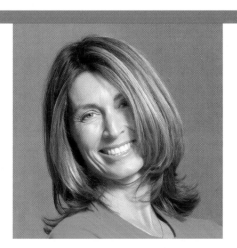

If you measure Yang Moderate or 6 on the Element Barometer, you need to introduce Water to your lifestyle and your appearance. By taking sacred steps and adding a Water cut or color, you can eliminate the totally structured look of Metal by adding chic energy to the style. Water is used to diminish the rigid structure of Metal. Add Water to your life by spending an evening alone: just you, a good book, a cup of tea, and no time clock. You want to honor the Metal/Earth element, but you want to add more sass to your style.

Haircut to Harmonize Metal/Earth 6

Harmonize with Water by rounding and softening layers to create dance within the hair. You are looking for a flirty style with boundaries. Use styling products to create kick or movement within the haircut. Refer to Chapter 11: Hairstyling for Your Body Type, Face Shape, and Facial Features for the best haircut and length.

Hair color to Harmonize Metal/Earth 6

Add Water element to your hair color by referring to Chapter 12: Skin Tone and Hair Color for your color selection. If you are a natural level six, you may select from levels two through five or seven through eleven. This is a wide range of colors. It is most important that you are absolutely positive about your skin tone when selecting a color. Refer to Chapter 11: Hairstyling for Your Body Type, Face Shape, and Facial Features for highlighting placement application and techniques. Water element will add a more sensual look to the style.

Balance Metal/Earth 8

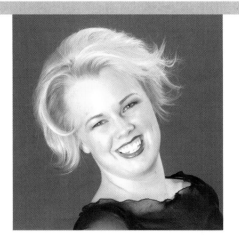

If you measured Yang Extreme or 8 on the Element Barometer, you have too much Metal or structure and need to be balanced. Adding Fire to Metal makes it more pliable and productive. Fire enables Metal to become more expressive and creative. Introduce Fire into your life by taking dance lessons or by changing the colors in your home to make it more expressive. Add bold colors in your wardrobe or bold accessories. In your appearance, I recommend a gradual makeover. You need to be ready to take the risk and be ready for the change in your life. The change has to come from inside as well as outside in order for you to be in balance.

Haircut to Balance Metal/Earth 8

Balance with Fire by adding uneven texture to create a bolder look. Your goal is a more expressive and freer hairstyle. Refer to Chapter 11: Hairstyling for Your Body Type, Face Shape, and Facial Features for the best haircut and length for you. Your goal is to unleash your hidden creativity and let it shine through a sensational haircut.

Hair color to Balance Metal/Earth 8

Balance with Fire by creating fun pieces of color. Refer to Chapter 12: Skin Tone and Hair Color before selecting the best colors for you. With the Fire element, you may select any color as long as it matches your skin tone. I recommend you take sacred steps before drastically changing your hair color. Make certain that you are ready inside to accept the change. Refer to Chapter 11: Hairstyling for Your Body Type, Face Shape, and Facial Features for highlighting techniques and placement. I would recommend balancing with a Fire cut, highlighting, or color, not all at once.

Metal/Metal

Metal/Metal types love detail and the opportunity to make the best better. Metal/Metal types are excellent at research and creating innovative technology. If your car isn't running smoothly or you have a glitch with your computer, a Metal/Metal friend is the one to have. Their emotions are not easily revealed as they won't let you get too close to them. They love luxurious objects and thrive on the most expensive or sought-after piece of art. Metal/Metal types are not considered to be the romantic types who will sweep you off your feet while whispering sweet nothings in your ear. They are, however, the reliable ones that you can count on to remember your anniversary or birthday. An attorney or accountant who is Metal/Metal will know all of the laws pertaining to your company. They can be *too* focused, which can create health issues. They are very driven to excel. Sometimes they get sidetracked on small details and do not reach their ultimate potential. They can be the ones who pick lint off your sweater while ignoring what you say. They have the ability to be totally lost in concentration and not in the moment. They would never follow the latest fad or fashion in clothing. Their fashion style can be described as classic or traditional. Think of a tweed coat for a male and a Chanel suit for a female.

Harmonize Metal/Metal 2

If you measure Yin Extreme or 2 on the Element Barometer, you need to add the Earth influence, as you have a deficiency of Metal in your life, attitude, and appearance. Earth creates Metal. I recommend taking sacred steps to stabilize your Metal element. Spend some time working on your lawn or planting a garden. Volunteer for the Boys and Girls Club or the YMCA. Earth types are very caring and nurturing as they focus on others instead of themselves. Metal types become focused on their profession and forget the world around them. Adding the Earth element will solidify the Metal element.

Haircut to Harmonize Metal/Metal 2
Harmonize with Earth by using the softening shear to support the natural style without destroying classic lines. Refer to Chapter 11: Hairstyling for Your Body Type, Face Shape, and Facial Features for the best haircut and length for you. You want a no-fuss, natural style that does not require a lot of styling time.

Hair color to Harmonize Metal/Metal 2
Harmonize with Earth by referring to Chapter 12: Skin Tone and Hair Color for your color selection. If you are a natural level four, you may select colors from

levels two or three, or five or six. Refer to Chapter 11: Hairstyling for Your Body Type, Face Shape, and Facial Features for highlighting placement, application, and techniques. The goal is to have a softer, more natural sun-kissed highlighting.

Enhance Metal/Metal 4

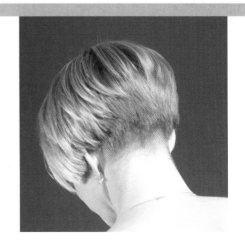

If you measure Yin Moderate or 4, you need to add more structure to your look. You see yourself as disciplined and focused, but your look does not provide an accurate reflection. I recommend adding Metal in your cut and color for a more classic look. This may result in quite a change, but one that will be very satisfying as it will reflect who you are.

Haircut to Enhance Metal/Metal 4
Enhance with Metal, creating sharp classic lines with no disarray. The perfect cut will create a more professional, elegant style that is timeless. Refer to Chapter 11: Hairstyling for Your Body Type, Face Shape, and Facial Features for the best hair cut and length. You want a precision cut that is impeccable and classic.

Hair color to Enhance Metal/Metal 4
Enhance with Metal by turning to Chapter 12 for the correct colors for you. If you are a natural level six, you may select colors from levels three through five or seven through ten. Refer to Chapter 11: Hairstyling for Your Body Type, Face Shape, and Facial Features for highlighting placement for your face shape and techniques. You want an elegant color that looks as though you were born with the perfect color and nature created the perfect variances of color in your hair—which we call highlights.

Harmonize Metal/Metal 6

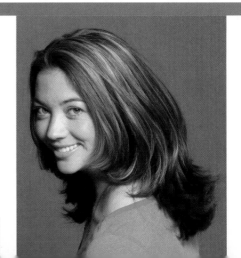

If you measure Yang Moderate or 6 on the Element Barometer, you need to add Water to create more pizzazz in your style. Water flows and is great for encouraging freedom in someone who is too structured. Metal types sometimes become so focused on the task at hand that they forget to think about the future. Water types are visionaries and more concerned about what lies ahead. They are open to change and are excited about new opportunities. By adding Water to your life and your appearance, you open new opportunities for growth.

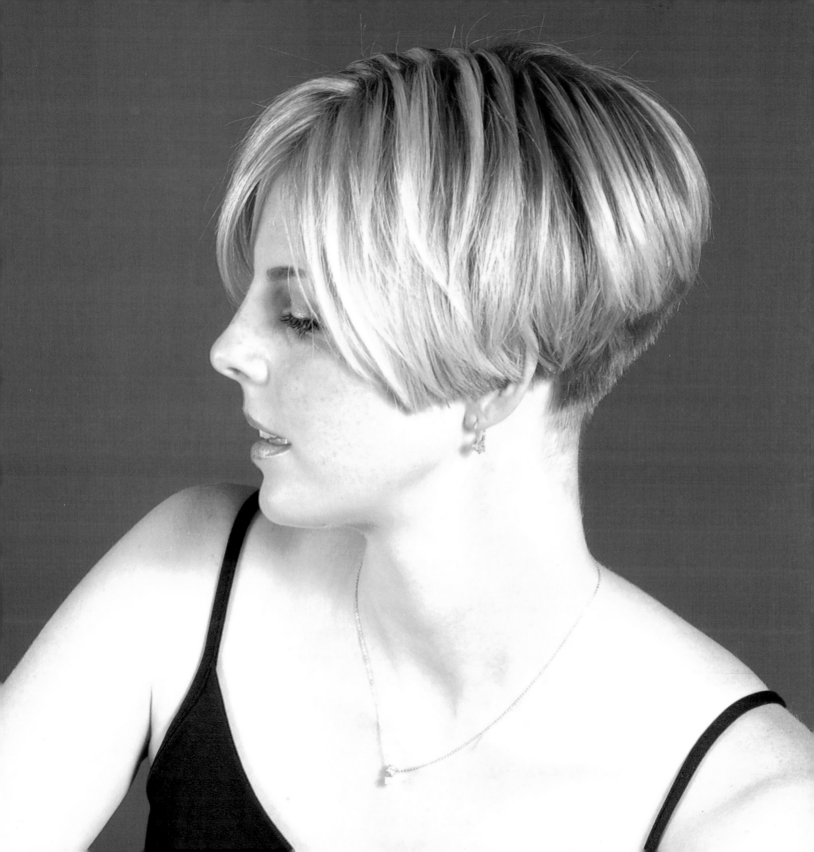

Haircut to Harmonize Metal/Metal 6

Harmonize with Water to create a sophisticated, sassy-flirty attitude. Let texture create the kick. Refer to Chapter 11: Hairstyling for Your Body Type, Face Shape, and Facial Features for the best haircut and length. You want a cut that is fashionable, yet sassy—a great combination that expresses excitement.

Hair color to Harmonize Metal/Metal 6

Harmonize with Water by referring to Chapter 12: Skin Tone and Hair Color for your color selection. The Water element offers a great variety of colors according to your skin tone. If you are a natural level seven, you may select colors from levels three through six or eight through eleven. Refer to Chapter 11: Hairstyling for Your Body Type, Face Shape, and Facial Features for your highlighting placement and techniques. Your color should have more excitement using these colors and techniques.

Balance Metal/Metal 8

If you measure Yang Extreme or 8 on the Element Barometer, you need to balance your look and life with Fire. Take sacred steps in adding Fire to your life. Begin with the addition of an artistic expression: singing, dancing, painting, playing a musical instrument, cooking, designing, or sewing. Write poetry that expresses your love and the joys you discover in your day. Do not select both a Fire cut and color, as Fire can be very explosive if out of control. Fire added gradually will cause the Metal/Metal type to become more expressive and open.

Haircut to Balance Metal/Metal 8

Balance with Fire by creating a disconnected and textured hairstyle that will be bold and expressive. Refer to Chapter 11: Hairstyling for Your Body Type, Face Shape, and Facial Features for the length and cut for you.. Be careful, as adding too much Fire will create a total makeover in your looks. If you are willing and feel that it is time for a change, then enjoy!

Hair color to Balance Metal/Metal 8

Balance with Fire by turning to Chapter 12: Skin Tone and Hair Color for color selection based on your skin tone and element. The only limitation you have when selecting a color is your skin tone. Be cautious as you want to take sacred steps in achieving balance. Refer to Chapter 11: Hairstyling for Your Body Type, Face Shape, and Facial Features for highlight placement application and techniques. You want an expressive look, but you must avoid too much flash.

Metal/Water

What a great combination! When in balance, the Metal/Water type is focused with a vision. They appear to be the most reliable ones who will work effortlessly to complete a project. Sometimes they take on too much as they don't like to say no when asked for help. They have the organizational skills to make a goal become a reality. If you are a Metal/Water type, you enjoy beautiful objects and are strongly attracted to being in love. You are aware when others dote on you and appreciate you as a friend. You can be temperamental if the rigidity of Metal combined with the fluidity of Water is not in balance.

You are blessed with a natural gift for negotiating and sharing your ideals with others. Metal/Water types have the ability to be great leaders. You focus on the future when making decisions.

Harmonize Metal/Water 2

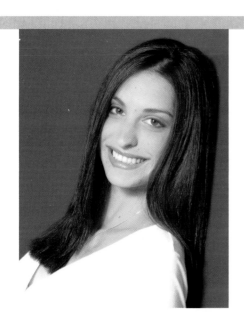

If you measure 2 on the Element Barometer, you need to add Earth to soften your life and appearance. Earth types are very stable and possess a great knowledge of the present. Their focus is on those around them and their environment, while Metal types are more focused on their career than those around them. By becoming involved in a community or charity organization, it lessens the focus on them and opens the opportunity to allow others to enter their lives. When adding Earth, it is important not to add too much, as you don't want to destroy the Metal, only soften it.

Haircut to Harmonize Metal/Water 2

Harmonize with Earth using texture for support, while still keeping the structure of Metal. Refer to Chapter 11: Hairstyling for Your Body Type, Face Shape, and Facial Features for the best length and haircut. Earth cuts are usually very natural with a clean basic style. You don't want to eliminate the classic look of Metal, you only want to add a natural, organic look to the cut.

Hair color to Harmonize Metal/Water 2

Harmonize with Earth by referring to Chapter 12: Skin Tone and Hair Color for color selections according to your skin tone and element. If you are a natural level six in your hair color, you may select colors from levels four or five, or seven or eight. Refer to Chapter 11: Hairstyling for Your Body Type, Face Shape, and Facial Features for highlighting placement techniques. Too much Earth will destroy the structure of Metal, so take sacred steps in adding Earth.

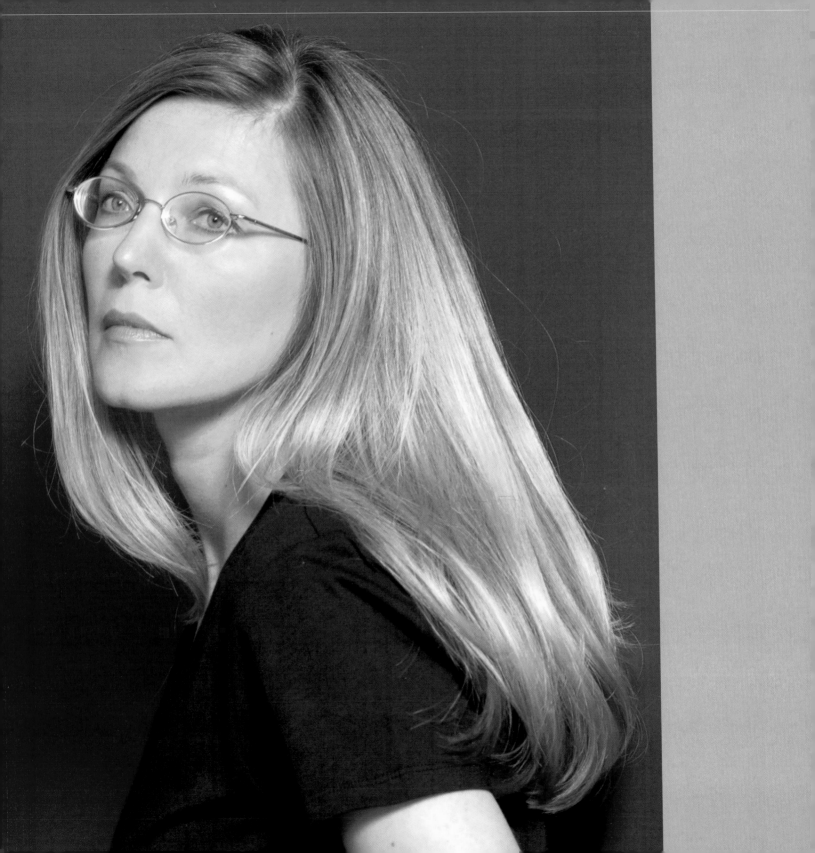

Enhance Metal/Water 4

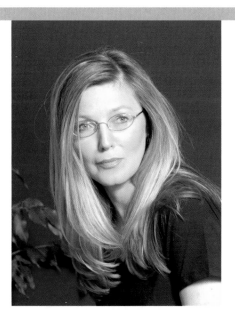

If you measure Yin Moderate or 4 on the Element Barometer, you need to add more Metal to your life. Metal will create more structure and allow you to become stronger and more focused. If you add too much Metal, you will become rigid and removed from your family and community. The key is to add more activities that involve your mental acuity and that allow you to participate with others, such as chess matches. If you add a Metal haircut, color, and highlights, your look will be structured.

Haircut to Enhance Metal/Water 4
Enhance with Metal to create a sensual style without a confined look—classic with freedom within the style. Refer to Chapter 11: Hairstyling for Your Body Type, Face Shape, and Facial Features for the best length and haircut. You want a classic style with sass.

Hair color to Enhance Metal/Water 4
Enhance with Metal color by referring to Chapter 12: Skin Tone and Hair Color for the list of colors according to your skin tone and element. If you are a natural level six, you may select colors from levels three through five or seven through ten. Refer to Chapter 11: Hairstyling for Your Body Type, Face Shape, and Facial Features for highlighting techniques and placement. You are striving for a classic look with your hair color.

Harmonize Metal/Water 6

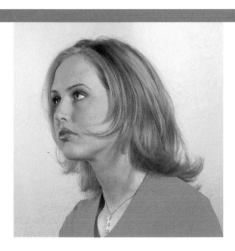

If you measure Yang Moderate or 6 on the Element Barometer, you need to add Water to create more expression and freedom. You have too much Metal in your life and appearance. Create a sensual, chic look. Add travel or reading to your life to open up new opportunities and knowledge.

Haircut to Harmonize Metal/Water 6
Harmonize with Water using texture to create a chic style that kicks. Refer to Chapter 11: Hairstyling for Your Body Type, Face Shape, and Facial Features for the best haircut and length. You want a free-flowing style that adds a lift or fashion with a twist.

Hair color to Harmonize Metal/Water 6
Use Water highlighting techniques. Try the more expressive ones that include

slicing in a brick pattern. Refer to Chapter 11: Hairstyling for Your Body Type, Face Shape, and Facial Features for highlights placement and techniques. Refer to Chapter 12: Skin Tone and Hair Color for the color selection listed according to your skin tone, hair level, and element. If you are a natural level five, you may select colors from levels one through four or six through ten. This is a wide range of colors so pay attention when making your selection. You may want to stay closer to your own natural level and then gradually introduce other colors. If you are willing to experiment, you may use demi-permanent colors until you find the ones you prefer.

Balance Metal/Water 8

If you measure Yang Extreme or 8 on the Element Barometer, you need to add Fire. Fire added to Metal/Water can be very exciting. The Metal/Water type is receptive to different techniques and even a complete makeover. Take steps to achieve the look you want and/or need to make a change in your appearance and life. Add some Fire to your lifestyle by getting involved in an artistic experience. You may want to begin by painting a room in a bright, expressive color or by changing your clothing style to show more expression. You be the judge as this is all about you.

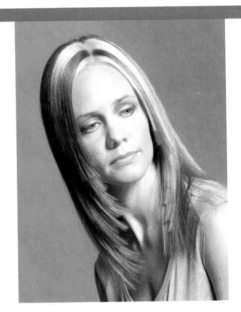

Haircut to Balance Metal/Water 8

Balance with Fire by adding disconnected, uneven pieces in a chic style. You want it to be expressive but not explosive. Refer to Chapter 11: Hairstyling for Your Body Type, Face Shape, and Facial Features for the best length and haircut. Be creative and have fun with your new look.

Hair color to Balance Metal/Water 8

Balance with Fire by using Fire highlighting techniques listed in Chapter 12: Skin Tone and Hair Color. You will find highlight placement according to face shape in Chapter 11: Hairstyling for Your Body Type, Face Shape, and Facial Features. Refer to Chapter 12 for the correct color for you. The only limitation is your skin tone; otherwise, you have total freedom in selecting any color. Allow yourself to enjoy the freedom of a new you. If you are hesitant, then use either the cut or the color.

Metal/Wood

Metal/Wood types love to entertain and be with others. They are the most fun-loving of the Metal types. They are optimistic and make good partners in business and in marriage. While disciplined and focused, they enjoy sharing information with others. They can be very influential if the elements are in balance. They dislike being alone, as they love sharing pleasures with others. A love of the outdoors means they often prefer a job that keeps them out of the office.

Metal/Wood types are great at communicating their ideas. As writers, they are focused, have the discipline for meeting deadlines, and can tell a story in an articulate manner. Metal/Wood types are great as war correspondents as they have the focus and discipline to stay on task while telling facts along with personal information about people or events. They love variety and are not content with following rituals or traditions.

Harmonize Metal/Wood 2

If you measure Yin Extreme or 2 on the Element Barometer, you need to add Earth. You will want to stabilize the Metal by creating warmth and a foundation. You may want to become involved as a Big Brother or Big Sister or volunteer at a shelter for women and children. You want to introduce a freer natural look without destroying the structure.

Haircut to Harmonize Metal/Wood 2

Harmonize with Earth by creating natural organic lines with loose styling within a traditional classic Metal cut. Refer to Chapter 11: Hairstyling for Your Body Type, Face Shape, and Facial Features for the best length and haircut.

Hair color to Harmonize Metal/Wood 2

Harmonize with Earth by referring to Chapter 12: Skin Tone and Hair Color for the color selection according to your skin tone and element. If you are a natural level eight, you may select colors from levels six or seven, or nine or ten. Refer to Chapter 11: Hairstyling for Your Body Type, Face Shape, and Facial Features for highlighting techniques. You will want Earth coloring techniques and colors; however, it is vital that you keep the colors rich.

Enhance Metal/Wood 4

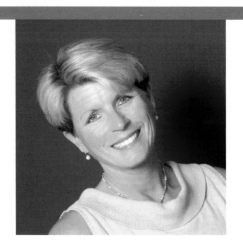

If you measure Yin Moderate or 4 on the Element Barometer, you need to add Metal element to enhance the Metal in your life and appearance. I recommend adding the Metal element to your life by organizing your room and your closet. Remove all of the magazines you have accumulated. Cut out the articles you want to save and immediately place them in a file. If you can't remember why you saved the magazine or newspaper, discard it. Free yourself of the clothes you have saved, waiting for the day when you could wear the dress with the tiny waist or waiting for your granny boots to come back into style. If you must save clothing from the important years of your life, place it into a plastic see-through storage box and label it.

When I reluctantly agreed to reduce my T-shirt collection, I found T-shirts that I had saved for no reason other than I had worn them. Some T-shirts marked momentous occasions in my life and were placed in the storage box. The better T-shirts were given to homeless shelters, and the soft, worn-out T-shirts with holes became dusting cloths or filled our garbage cans. This experience of paring down items was cleansing and encouraged me to allocate time weekly to organize my closet and garage. I carried this over to my office and to my life. I recommend adding the Metal element to your appearance as well as to your life.

Haircut to Enhance Metal/Wood 4

Enhance with Metal by selecting a style with texture for movement within structured lines. A precision haircut with meticulous styling definitely depicts a Metal. Refer to Chapter 11: Hairstyling for Your Body Type, Face Shape, and Facial Features for the best length and haircut. You want a classic Metal cut.

Hair color to Enhance Metal/Wood 4

Enhance with Metal by referring to Chapter 12: Skin Tone and Hair Color for your color selection. If you are a natural level four, you may select colors from levels one through three, or five through eight. Refer to Chapter 11: Hairstyling for Your Body Type, Face Shape, and Facial Features for highlight placement and techniques. You may use one to three colors in your highlights for a gradual variance of color. These highlights should be very thin and not obvious.

Harmonize Metal/Wood 6

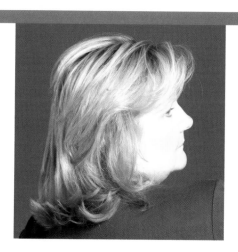

If you measure Yang Moderate or 6 on the Element Barometer, you need to add Water to break up the rigidity of Metal. You may add Water to your lifestyle by spending the evening at your favorite bookstore, curled up on the sofa reading, or enjoying the solitude of your home. A Water type is open to change and has a thirst for knowledge.

Haircut to Harmonize Metal/Wood 6

Harmonize with Water by adding sassy texture to the edges of classic lines. Make the cut more expressive as you also have the influence of Wood which needs a lot of movement within the cut. Refer to Chapter 11: Hairstyling for Your Body Type, Face Shape, and Facial Features for the best haircut and length. You want a flirty style that is still professional.

Hair color to Harmonize Metal/Wood 6

Harmonize with Water by referring to Chapter 12: Skin Tone and Hair Color for the correct colors according to your skin tone, natural hair color level, and element. If you are a natural level six, you may select from levels two through five, or seven through eleven. Refer to Chapter 11: Hairstyling for Your Body Type, Face Shape, and Facial Features for highlight placement, application, and highlighting techniques. Strive for a chic hair color.

Balance Metal/Wood 8

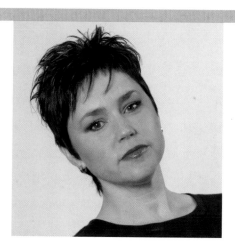

If you measure Yang Extreme or 8 on the Element Barometer, introduce Fire to your life for more brilliance and expression in your appearance. Add some excitement to your life by fulfilling a long-forgotten dream. Remember the passion you had about sailing around the world or spending a summer in a foreign land. The dream was put on a shelf while you went about the daily task of living and being responsible. Now is the time for you to seek the excitement that you felt when you thought or talked about what you would do if... The amount of Fire element you add to your life and your appearance depends on you. You are in the driver's seat and determine the degree of change.

Haircut to Balance Metal/Wood 8

Balance with Fire by creating uneven pieces for a kicky, free style. Refer to Chapter 11: Hairstyling for Your Body Type, Face Shape, and Facial Features for your best length and cut. A cut that is bold and expressive without being chaotic would work for you.

Hair color to Balance Metal/Wood 8

Balance with Fire by using fun highlighting techniques and bold, expressive colors. Refer to Chapter 12: Skin Tone and Hair Color for your color selection according to skin tone and element. Your skin tone will determine the color; with Fire you may select from the whole rainbow of colors. Refer to Chapter 11: Hairstyling for Your Body Type, Face Shape, and Facial Features for highlight placement and application, as well as highlighting techniques. With the Fire element, you set the limits.

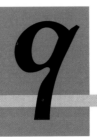 # Water Element

When water is free-flowing, it brings life and vitality to its surroundings. A clear mountain stream can meander or flow rapidly, depending on the obstacles in its way. When water is stagnant it becomes dark and smelly. Fish and plants die and the water becomes toxic. The deeper the water, the slower it flows. The same is true with people who are the Water type. They tend to be reflective, and meditate to keep in balance. Water types can be influenced by other people as well as the boundaries they set on their own. Just as water flows forward, Water types are visionaries. They are always seeking ways to improve themselves. Look for them in the self-help section at your local bookstore. It is important for Water types to be balanced, as too much or too little Water can be destructive. Think of a flood or a drought and the damage that is done to the environment when either one occurs. Water types are apt to listen deeply and think about what is being said to them. They are able to hear and understand both sides of an issue.

Water types love to read about a wide spectrum of subjects. They become absorbed in a book and are unaware of others around them. It is not unusual for Water people to read or listen to numerous books at one time and keep the content separate in their mind. They are rarely in the Now, because they are busy thinking about an idea for a new venture. If you need someone to give you ideas for decorating, call a Water friend. They won't have time to help you, but they will take the time to share their pearls of wisdom with you. Too much reading means that not enough of the information becomes a reality, so Water types need to keep active.

Water types make lasting friends, although their list of friends is not long. It is not unusual for their group to include childhood friends. They have great instincts and when they don't follow them, it leads to disaster. Water types are secretive and don't like for others to intrude on their space. They expect others to respect their need for privacy.

When Water types are in balance, they light up a room and own the audience. When Water types are out of balance, they tend to overreact rather than listen and then act. They don't like to be challenged, as they are usually sure of their information before they speak.

Water types express their flair in choices of clothing and accessories. Although they are always chic, they are willing to wear designer clothing that is a little on the edge. Their sense of style is impeccable, and they are able to appear fashionable even on casual occasions. They are rarely true to any one designer, but prefer an eclectic range of styles.

Within each element, Yin and Yang energies exist. On the Element Barometer, I have listed characteristics that will assist you in knowing whether you need to enhance, harmonize or balance the element. If the Water element is hidden or Yin Extreme 2, you need to harmonize by adding Metal element to encourage more structure. When the Yin is moderate 4, you need to enhance the Water by adding more Water. If the Yang is moderate 6, reduce the Water by adding Wood to absorb the Water. If the Yang is extreme 8, Earth is needed to balance the rushing Water. The intensity of the Water can be compared to the movement of water in our world. A tidal wave that wreaks havoc upon everything in its way can be contained with the addition of Earth. This tidal wave is similar to Yang Extreme 8 on the Element Barometer. Yang Moderate 6 is similar to a river overflowing its banks during heavy rains, and needs Wood to stop or slow the Water. Yin Water 2 is stagnant or still water that needs more Water to get it moving.

Using Feng Shui principles designed to bring balance and create a flow of good Chi, I take into consideration not only your haircut, hair color, makeup, body type, and face shape, but also your hobbies, lifestyle, exercise patterns, meditation habits, clothing, and accessories. All of these things affect you and the image you portray. When I prescribe the look that will best reflect how you perceive yourself, I also address the other factors that influence your life. Some of the changes or recommendations will be evident immediately such as haircut, hair color, and makeup. The other changes involve more participation from you and will evolve, as you are the one in charge of implementing that part of your life. The amount of change will depend upon your dedication.

Makeup for the Water Element

Just as water flows, moves, and changes, a Water element person is willing to change hairstyles, cuts, colors, and makeup. Since they like to be fashionable, they are ready to change with the times. A Water person will adjust makeup styles according to seasons and the time of day. In the evening, the makeup will appear more dramatic.

Makeup is a beautiful way to emphasize your expressive eyes, your classic cheekbones, or your luscious full lips. Applying makeup flawlessly requires experience and patience. You can have fun trying new looks by selecting strong colors for your eyes and/or lips. You want a chic, sophisticated look with a dash of sass.

Porcelain
Try bone white, pink, lavender, light blue, or blue gray eye shadows, eyes lined with gray blue, and nude to pink gloss on lips.

Milky
Try charcoal-lined eyes with peach or warm brown eye shadow, and peach to nude to rust shades on lips.

Honey
Use smoky brown eyeliner with rust and gold eye shadows, and red-orange on lips.

Olive
Apply black or gray eyeliner with berry or burgundy eye shadows. Berry or deep red on lips.

Ebony
Apply strong colors on eyes and berry or russet browns on lips.

Ruby
Use flat browns, ivory, cream, and a hint of green on eyes, and brown to red-brown on lips.

Water/Fire

If you selected Water for your personality and Fire for your lifestyle, you're a walking contradiction. Water is reflective and likes to meditate, while Fire is active and reacts to situations instantly. It takes time for these types to come to terms with their emotions. They often are entertainers and come alive on the stage or in front of a crowd. That way they can keep others at arm's length and avoid sharing any intimate information. Water/Fire types can be hard to understand; just when you think you have them pegged, they show you a different side. Their mystique intrigues those who come under their spell. It is hard to change their opinions; usually you have to present your case and give them time. Eventually, they will think it is their idea and will welcome it. A Water/Fire type may present a chic appearance during the day at work, but at night, the Fire element takes over and they become the life of the party.

Water/Fire types spend hours perusing magazines for a look at the latest fashions or the newest designer. They want to be in the know about what is going on and what will be the look for the next season. They have exquisite taste for decorating and for fashion. Rather than deal with mundane issues that arise daily, they will retreat to their own world. They delegate trivial problems to others; personal issues or shortcomings are a source of irritation.

Water/Fire types make dynamic speakers. They have the passion of the Fire element and the drive to acquire thorough knowledge of their subject. They are great at motivating a large crowd—their energy will keep the audience on the edge of their seats. No one would dare to fall asleep as the message and delivery of the speech is electric.

Water types are usually reflective and it takes a long time for them to make decisions. Water/Fire types play it by intuition and can make a rapid decision without hesitating. Don't expect them to balance their checkbook or harness their shopping sprees—they display a total lack of concern about money. Money is never the driving force. As business owners, they will contribute energy, vision, and splendid taste to the organization. It behooves the Water/Fire type to hire Metal types to take care of the details of running the business, which frees them to do what they do best.

Harmonize Water/Fire 2

If you measure Yin Moderate or 2 on the Element Barometer, you need to add Metal to give Water more control and focus. Water/Fire types have no shortage of great ideas, but they lack the structure or focus for implementation.

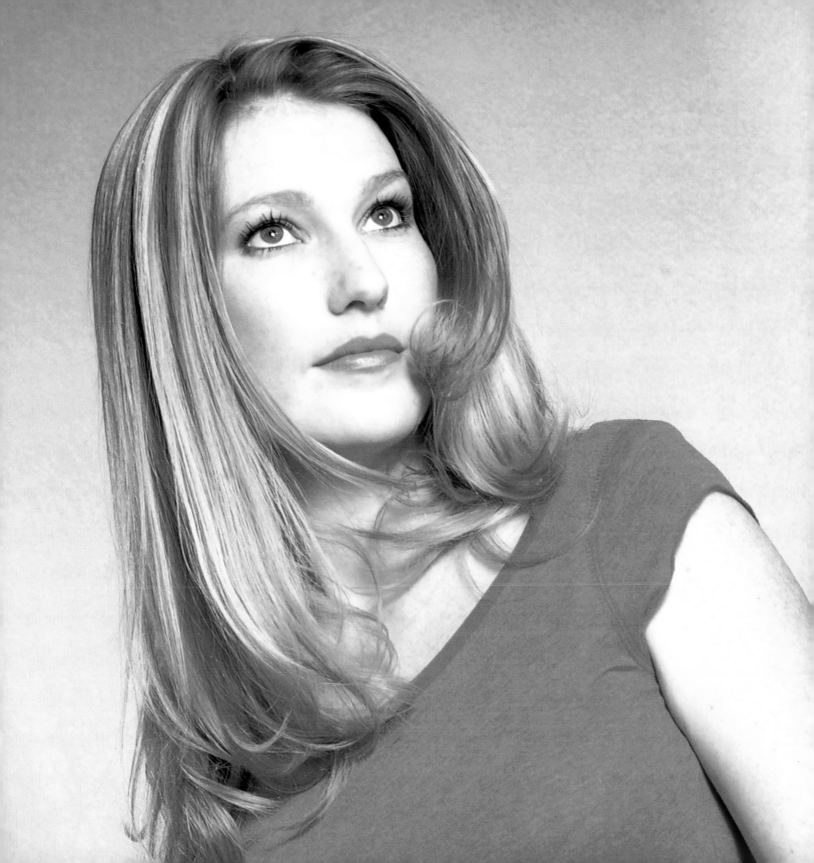

Metal contains Water and through condensation produces Water. Metal types are disciplined and efficient in all aspects of their life. I recommend Water/Fire types make a list each day of the tasks that need to be completed. Visiting this list several times during the day to make certain they are on track will help them to become more productive.

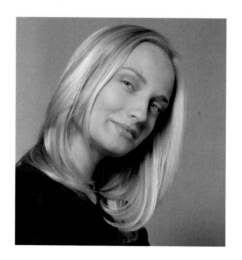

Haircut to Harmonize Water/Fire 2

Harmonize with Metal for a refined, flirty cut with texture. Look for a clean, sleek style for your hair. Think of a precision cut that has movement. Refer to Chapter 11: Hairstyling for Your Body Type, Face Shape, and Facial Features for the best length and cut. You are striving for a chic look with sass.

Hair color to Harmonize Water/Fire 2

Harmonize with Metal by following the color selections in Chapter 12: Skin Tone and Hair Color. Turn to the element section for your skin tone. If you are a natural level six, you may select colors from level three through five or seven through ten. For highlighting placement and techniques, refer to Chapter 11: Hairstyling for Your Body Type, Face Shape, and Facial Features. With highlights you may use one to three colors within the same color family. Metal highlights will be precise, with seven to nine pieces per pickup.

Enhance Water/Fire 4

If you measure Yin Moderate or 4 on the Element Barometer, you need to add more Water. Be careful when adding Water, as too much can be damaging, especially if the Water is not moving. You can enhance your lifestyle by enrolling in a night class at a local college or attending a motivational seminar.

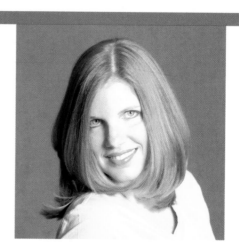

Haircut to Enhance Water/Fire 4

Enhance with Water by adding texture for dancing movement that creates sensual lines. You want a very feminine look with pizzazz. Refer to Chapter 11: Hairstyling for Your Body Type, Face Shape, and Facial Features for your best length and cut. I recommend a cut that is textured at the ends for a kick. You may want to cut into your hair for movement around your face, depending on your face shape.

Hair color to Enhance Water/Fire 4

Enhance with Water by using slicing in a brick pattern. Use one to three colors in your highlights for depth and variance. Refer to Chapter 12: Skin Tone and Hair Color for color selection. If your hair color is a natural level five, you may select colors from levels one through four or six through ten. A wide array of colors will work for Water types. Select a color you feel comfortable wearing. If you are unsure about making a drastic change, select a semi-permanent color at first.

Harmonize Water/Fire 6

If you measure Yang Moderate or 6 on the Element Barometer, you need to add Wood to slow down or redirect too much Water. Wood types are very outgoing and social. Too much Water causes people to be very reflective and moody. Join a gym, enroll in a dance class, or become involved with a civic organization. If you have children in school, volunteer to showcase your talent or to share information about your favorite author or book. In your appearance, I recommend creating movement for an active, tousled look.

Haircut to Harmonize Water/Fire 6
Harmonize with Wood, creating tousled, unstructured, jagged pieces in the style. Wood needs movement in order to flourish. Refer to Chapter 11: Hairstyling for Your Body Type, Face Shape, and Facial Features for the best length and cut. You want a hairstyle that can look wind-blown and still be professional when you need it. If you have curly hair, this is a great cut for you, as it will give your curls spring and movement. If you have longer hair, rounded layers will give you movement with sass.

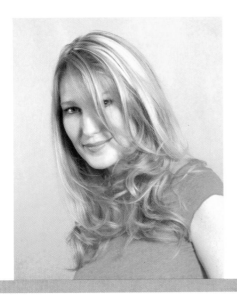

Hair color to Harmonize Water/Fire 6
Harmonize with Wood colors by referring to Chapter 12: Skin Tone and Hair Color for color selection based on your natural hair level, skin tone, and element. If you are a natural level seven, you may select colors from levels five or six, or eight through ten. Refer to Chapter 11: Hairstyling for Your Body Type, Face Shape, and Facial Features for highlighting placement and techniques. Use two to three colors for depth in your highlights.

Balance Water/Fire 8

If you measure Yang Extreme or 8 on the Element Barometer, you need to add Earth to diminish the flow of Water. Too much Water can be balanced or stopped with Earth. An Earth dam contains and controls Water. To add Earth to your life, volunteer at your children's school, the YMCA, or the Boys and Girls Club. Get involved with helping others. Plant a garden of flowers or vegetables and share your bounty with older friends who have difficulty working in the yard. In your appearance, the emphasis will be on a natural, organic look.

Haircut to Balance Water/Fire 8

Balance with Earth by adding soft texture for movement. Use softening shears on the ends for movement. Refer to Chapter 11: Hairstyling for Your Body Type, Face Shape, and Facial Features for the best length and cut. You want a natural look without having to spend a lot of time on the style.

Hair color to Balance Water/Fire 8

Balance with Earth by referring to Chapter 12: Skin Tone and Hair Color for color selections according to your skin tone, elements, and natural hair color level. If you are a natural level six, you may select colors from levels four or five, or seven or eight. Refer to Chapter 11: Hairstyling for Your Body Type, Face Shape, and Facial Features for highlighting techniques and placement. For Earth highlighting techniques, use four to six pieces per pickup for a natural, sun-kissed effect. Use two to three different colors from the same color family.

Water/Earth

The Water type is forward-moving and future-oriented, while the Earth type is in the moment. When in balance, this combination is productive and consistent. When not in balance, this type can easily be depleted, as they are not apt to take care of themselves. They make dependable and deeply caring friends, although they like to be alone and, even in a crowd, often appear aloof. They have a wide array of information at their disposal, but only close friends are privy to hearing it. They enjoy great stories and have a good sense of humor.

Water/Earth types dress very fashionably. Unlike Fire types, they will not select something just because it is the latest fad. They are concerned with their appearance and present a chic, professional image at work. Their hairstyle and makeup changes frequently; however, it is always very flattering. They will not try the latest cut unless they are confident that it suits their style. Their personality is more subdued than most Water types, and they are more genuinely empathetic with their friends and coworkers. They make great parents, putting their children's needs above theirs and even adjusting their work schedules around their children whenever it is feasible. They may become moody or quiet

when faced with problems and be unwilling to discuss them with others. They are loyal employees.

Harmonize Water/Earth 2

If you measure Yin Extreme or 2 on the Element Barometer, you need to add Metal to contain the Water. Water Yin Extreme 2 types are free-flowing, without boundaries—think of a glass of water spilled on the table or floor. Without boundaries, there is no energy and the Water becomes unusable and nonproductive. Metal types are focused, disciplined, and efficient. With the addition of Metal, Water/Earth types become more productive with increased energy.

Haircut to Harmonize Water/Earth 2

Harmonize with Metal by using clean, classic, soft lines in your haircut. The goal is to achieve a precision cut, but still keep a chic, sassy style. Refer to Chapter 11: Hairstyling for Your Body Type, Face Shape, and Facial Features for your best length and cut. If your hair is curly, you may want to use a flat iron or blow-dryer on your hair to straighten it for a sleek style. It is entirely up to you how much Metal element you wish to add.

Hair color to Harmonize Water/Earth 2

Harmonize with Metal by using the color selections in Chapter 12: Skin Tone and Hair Color. Be careful in identifying your skin tone, remembering that it will change with sun exposure. The colors are listed according to your skin tone, element, and natural color level. If you are a natural level six, you may select colors from levels three through five or seven through ten. Refer to Chapter 11: Hairstyling for Your Body Type, Face Shape, and Facial Features for highlighting placement and techniques. Use classic, refined Metal highlighting techniques.

Enhance Water/Earth 4

If you measure Yin Moderate or 4 on the Element Barometer, your Water element needs refilling with more Water. A Water type may become too emotional and unsure of her opinions. Set aside some time for you to meditate or reflect on your life. Browse in a bookstore and find a book about spirituality or self-improvement. Enroll in a yoga class. In beauty, I recommend adding more sass and chic in your look.

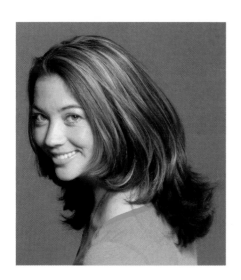

Haircut to Enhance Water/Earth 4

Enhance with Water by adding natural, gentle layering to create movement without restricting styling. Refer to Chapter 11: Hairstyling for Your Body Type, Face Shape, and Facial Features for the best length and cut. You want a demure yet flirty look.

Hair color to Enhance Water/Earth 4

Enhance with Water by selecting colors from Chapter 12: Skin Tone and Hair Color according to your natural hair color, skin tone, and element. If you are a natural level six, you may select colors from levels two through five or seven through eleven. Any of these colors will look good with your skin tone. It is up to you to determine how daring you want to be. Refer to Chapter 11: Hairstyling for Your Body Type, Face Shape, and Facial Features for highlighting placement and techniques.

Harmonize Water/Earth 6

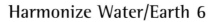

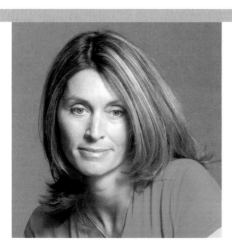

If you measure Yang Moderate or 6 on the Element Barometer, you need to reduce the amount of Water or slow it down. I recommend adding Wood element to harmonize. Join a gym or consult a personal trainer or industry professional for nutrition and exercise regimens. Become involved with the local theatre or go for a brisk walk with friends. You want to become more socially involved and have an evening of just fun, whether it's riding the roller coaster and screaming all the way down or going out dancing with a loved one. In beauty, I look for more movement and more freedom in the style.

Haircut to Harmonize Water/Earth 6

Harmonize with Wood to create soft, natural lines with flirty movement. Add texture to the ends for movement. If you prefer longer hair, adding rounded layers will add movement throughout the hair. Refer to Chapter 11: Hairstyling for Your Body Type, Face Shape, and Facial Features for the best length and haircut. The key to this cut is movement. Whether your hair is short or long, it should have a tousled look.

Hair color to Harmonize Water/Earth 6

Harmonize with the Wood colors shown in Chapter 12: Skin Tone and Hair Color. Colors are listed according to your skin tone, element, and natural color level. If you are a natural level seven, you may select colors from levels five or six, or eight through ten. For highlighting placement and techniques, refer to Chapter 11: Hairstyling for Your Body Type, Face Shape, and Facial Features.

Balance Water/Earth 8

Water element is concerned with the future and Water types often serve as the visionary in a business or home. If you measure Yang Extreme or 8 on the Element Barometer, you have too much Water and need to control it by adding the Earth element. Earth element is very nurturing and focused on the now. By adding Earth to your appearance, you will soften the look and make it more natural.

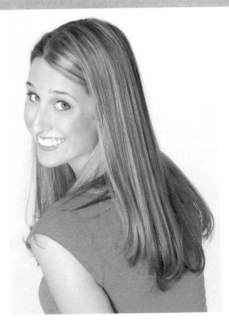

Haircut to Balance Water/Earth 8

Balance with Earth by creating a blunt cut with softening on the ends for a kick. You want very soft texture that has a natural look. Refer to Chapter 11: Hairstyling for Your Body Type, Face Shape, and Facial Features for the best length and cut. You want a look with style that will also honor your dominant Water element.

Hair color to Balance Water/Earth 8

Balance with Earth by referring to Chapter 12: Skin Tone and Hair Color for color selections based on your skin tone, element, and natural hair color level. If you are a natural level six, you may select colors from levels four or five, or seven or eight. Refer to Chapter 11: Hairstyling for Your Body Type, Face Shape, and Facial Features for highlighting techniques and placement. I would balance using Earth techniques and Water color selections, or Water techniques and Earth color selections. Don't add *too* much Earth, as it can destroy Water. You don't want to dam the Water element, you only want to channel it for good energy.

Water/Metal

Water/Metal types are persistent and can be very stubborn. The Water element seeks knowledge and dislikes being harnessed by others. The Metal element is detail-oriented and very focused on issues at hand. A type that combines these two elements can be quite successful in business—they research information and pay attention to the bottom line while planning for the future. They dislike friction and will avoid it at all cost, sometimes to their detriment. Too much Water can rust the Metal and too much Metal restricts the Water. The secret to creating good Chi or energy is to have the Water/Metal type in complete balance.

Water/Metal types spend time contemplating their decisions about the least situation. They are apt to work far into the night, having procrastinated and waited until the last minute to complete their projects. When finished, the results will be perfect and brilliant. Water/Metal types have a drive to know the latest information and put this information into their vision for a new project. They often have too many things going on at once, as everything sounds exciting and they hate to pass up any opportunity. They have a drive to excel and are their own worst enemy. When they are in balance, they are an asset to any company, and make great friends.

Harmonize Water/Metal 2

If you measure Yin Extreme or 2 on the Element Barometer, you need to introduce Metal into your life and your look. The Metal element creates Water by condensation and also holds Water. It is the support and structure the Water element needs. I recommend you take steps to organize your life, beginning with your closet, your room, and your home. You want to clear the clutter out of your life and have discipline to put your vision into action. I want to see more structure in your haircut and a refined look in your color. Be careful of adding too much Metal, as it contains Water and can quell its energy.

Haircut to Harmonize Water/Metal 2

Harmonize with Metal to create a chic, but classic, cut and attitude. You want to keep classic lines but achieve a flirty style. Refer to Chapter 11: Hairstyling for Your Body Type, Face Shape, and Facial Features for the best length and cut. It is important that you do not have a precision haircut, but rather one that has sleek, sharp lines.

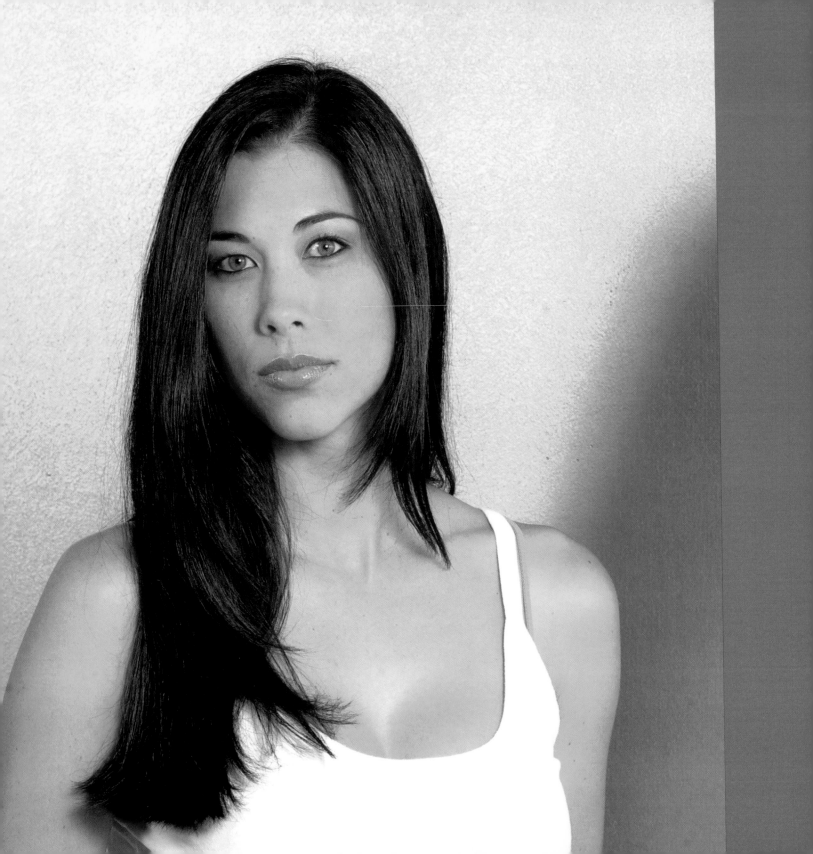

Hair color to Harmonize Water/Metal 2

Harmonize with Metal by referring to Chapter 12: Skin Tone and Hair Color for color selections based on your skin tone, natural hair color, and element. If you are a natural level six, you may select colors from levels three through five or seven through ten. Refer to Chapter 11: Hairstyling for Your Body Type, Face Shape, and Facial Features for highlighting placement and techniques. You are striving for very fine highlights.

Enhance Water/Metal 4

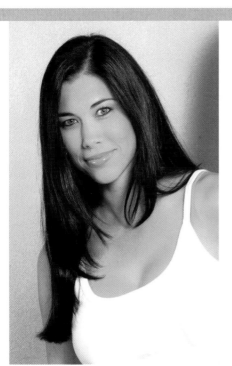

If you measure Yin Moderate or 4 on the Element Barometer, you need to refill your Water as your appearance and life do not reflect your element. Spend more time reading and planning for the future. Learn chess or have a rousing debate with a friend. In your appearance, I want to see more flirt and sass.

Haircut to Enhance Water/Metal 4

Enhance with Water, creating a chic, classic cut without confined structure. Cut into the classic cut to create movement. Refer to Chapter 11: Hairstyling for Your Body Type, Face Shape, and Facial Features for the best length and cut. If you have curly hair, you may want to straighten it with a flat iron and cut into the edges to create a kick.

Hair color to Enhance Water/Metal 4

Enhance with Water by referring to Chapter 12: Skin Tone and Hair Color for color selection and techniques based on your skin tone, element, and natural hair color level. If you are a natural level six, you may select colors from levels two through five or seven through eleven. Remember that too much Water can damage Metal so use either Water techniques or color, not both. For instance, if you choose a Water color, use Metal techniques. Refer to Chapter 11: Hairstyling for Your Body Type, Face Shape, and Facial Features for highlighting techniques and placement.

Harmonize Water/Metal 6

If you measure Yang Moderate or 6 on the Element Barometer, your Water element is out of control and needs to be reigned in by adding Wood. Wood will slow down the Water without eliminating its energy. Add an activity to your life that allows you to be involved with others, preferably outdoors. In beauty,

I am looking to add more movement to your cut and more energy to your color with highlighting techniques.

Haircut to Harmonize Water/Metal 6

Harmonize with Wood by creating a chic look with texture that allows movement. You can achieve this look by creating round layers in longer styles. For shorter styles, add texture and movement by cutting into the hair. This will give a springy look to curly hair for a flirty style.

Hair color to Harmonize Water/Metal 6

Harmonize with Wood by selecting colors from Chapter 12: Skin Tone and Hair Color. Color selections are based on your skin tone, element, and natural hair level. If you are a natural level five, you may select colors from levels three or four, or six through eight. Refer to Chapter 11: Hairstyling for Your Body Type, Face Shape, and Facial Features for highlighting placement and techniques. I recommend Wood highlights that have two to four pieces per pickup. This allows for more color, as the pieces are bigger. It will have a sporty, less sophisticated effect. You want to break up the Water, not stop it.

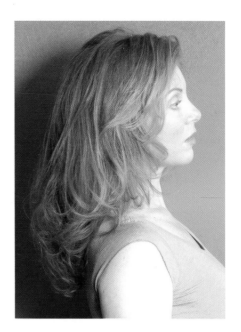

Balance Water/Metal 8

If you measure Yang Extreme or 8 on the Element barometer, your Water needs to be controlled by adding Earth. You want to control the Water, not stop it. When you have too much Water, you can become temperamental, secretive, and self-indulgent. Earth types are nurturing, patient, and very concerned for those around them. I recommend that you volunteer with your children's school, the Girls and Boys Club, a senior citizens' home, or another worthy cause. For your appearance, I am looking to add a natural, organic look with chic styling.

Haircut to Balance Water/Metal 8

Balance with Earth for a soft, semi-classic style. You may prefer a one-length cut that offers many styling opportunities. The look should require little styling time and still look chic. Refer to Chapter 11: Hairstyling for Your Body Type, Face Shape, and Facial Features for the best length and cut for you.

Hair color to Balance Water/Metal 8

Balance with Earth colors by referring to Chapter 12: Skin Tone and Hair Color for color selection and techniques. The colors are based on your skin tone, natural hair color level, and element. If you are a natural level five, you may select colors from levels three or four, or six or seven. I would select either Earth techniques or color, not both, and use Water for the other selection. Refer to Chapter 11: Hairstyling for Your Body Type, Face Shape, and Facial Features for highlighting placement and techniques.

Water/Water

There is no going halfway with Water/Water types. They love, hate, fight, cry, and hurt intensely. They listen intently, but they are not apt to move quickly. If you need to make a decision quickly, don't ask a Water/Water type for help. They need to consider all possible aspects of the situation and can become almost paralyzed with decision making. Choosing a frame and mat for a painting can take hours for a Water/Water type, and even then, they are not certain that it's the best one. Too much thinking and reflection can keep the best ideas from becoming realities. The Water type is by nature very sensual, but this sensuality can become hidden with too much Water.

Water/Water types have an innate sense of style and are able to mix and match accessories for a chic appearance. They are usually quiet and reserved without being cold. They have a thirst for knowledge and are eager to read the latest book. They have a wide range of interests. They are fun-loving and enjoy activities that do not necessarily involve others, but are loyal and compassionate with their chosen friends. The goal is to find a balance to create good energy with Water/Water.

Harmonize Water/Water 2

If you measure Yin Extreme or 2 on the Element Barometer, you need to add Metal. Metal offers shape to give the Water more energy. I recommend adding Metal to your lifestyle by focusing on your goals and designing a strategy to achieve them. In your appearance, I recommend adding a precise cut with a classic look.

Haircut to Harmonize Water/Water 2

Harmonize with Metal by getting a clean, symmetrical cut, keeping it professional and sassy. Refer to Chapter 11: Hairstyling for Your Body Type, Face Shape, and Facial Features for the best length and cut. You want a controlled, sassy look.

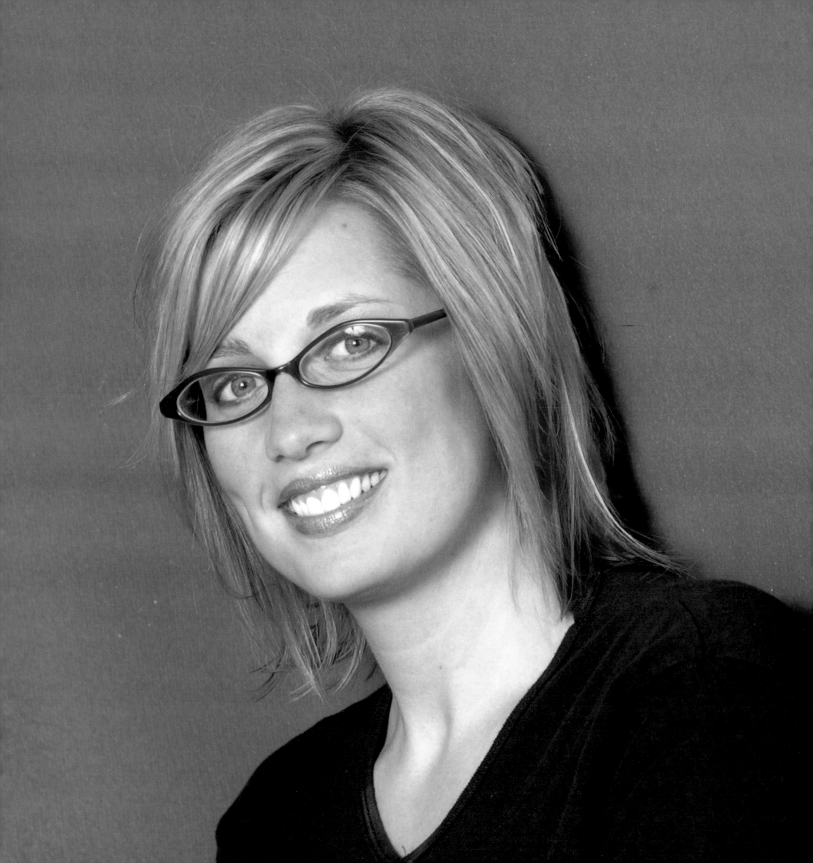

Hair color to Harmonize Water/Water 2

Harmonize with Metal by referring to Chapter 12: Skin Tone and Hair Color for color selections based on your skin tone, natural hair color, and element. If you are a natural level seven, you may select colors from levels four through six, or eight through eleven. Refer to Chapter 11: Hairstyling for Your Body Type, Face Shape, and Facial Features for highlighting placement and techniques. You want to create an elegant weave of color.

Enhance Water/Water 4

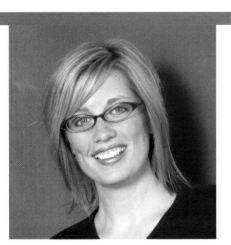

If you measure Yin Moderate or 4, you need to add Water to express the Water that is hidden. Add Water in your life by meditating and attending to your spiritual needs. Get to know yourself by keeping a journal or spending a day alone at a museum or art gallery. In adding more Water to your appearance, I am looking for a kicky, sassy, sophisticated style. You want a style that really expresses who you are inside.

Haircut to Enhance Water/Water 4

Enhance with Water, using notching shears to create movement with uneven, flirty lines—chic with a kick. Refer to Chapter 11: Hairstyling for Your Body Type, Face Shape, and Facial Features for the best length and cut. Look for an expressive hairstyle.

Hair color to Enhance Water/Water 4

Enhance with Water by using very sexy, classic colors from Chapter 12: Skin Tone and Hair Color. The color selection is based on your skin tone, natural hair color level, and element. Refer to Chapter 11: Hairstyling for Your Body Type, Face Shape, and Facial Features for highlighting placement and techniques. This is your opportunity to be expressive with your hair color and make it fit who you are.

Harmonize Water/Water 6

If you measure Yang Moderate or 6 on the Element Barometer, you need to introduce Wood element to your life and appearance. Wood will slow down the overabundance of Water element traits. You need to become more social and involved with others. Invite your friends for an afternoon at the beach or another fun place. I recommend adding Wood element to your hairstyle by adding a lot of movement and freedom in the cut and color.

Haircut to Harmonize Water/Water 6

Harmonize with Wood by creating texture from temples to the ends of your hair, rounded out following head shape. Refer to Chapter 11: Hairstyling for Your Body Type, Face Shape, and Facial Features for the best length and cut. You want a hairstyle that says you are always ready to go at a moment's notice.

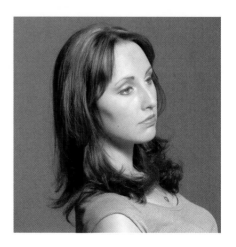

Hair color to Harmonize Water/Water 6

Harmonize with Wood by referring to Chapter 12: Skin Tone and Hair Color for color selections based on your skin tone, natural hair level, and element. If you are a natural level five, you may select colors from levels three or four, or six through eight. Refer to Chapter 11: Hairstyling for Your Body Type, Face Shape, and Facial Features for highlighting placement and techniques. You want to create more color with your highlights, with large sections of color and separation between highlights.

Balance Water/Water 8

If you measure Yang Extreme or 8 on the Element Barometer, you need to add Earth to balance or contain your out-of-control Water element. Spend some time with children; experience their joy and renew your appreciation of the world around you. Join a group to clean up the environment in your community. If no such group exists, start one. For your appearance, I recommend creating a more natural look in your haircut and color.

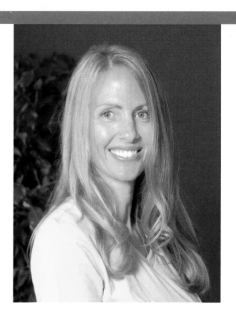

Haircut to Balance Water/Water 8

Balance with Earth to create a softer kick and less texture. Refer to Chapter 11: Hairstyling for Your Body Type, Face Shape, and Facial Features for the best length and cut. If your hair is curly, let it dry naturally. You want a style that has some texture in the cut for volume and to remove the weight, but to create a one-length effect.

Hair color to Balance Water/Water 8

Balance with Earth colors found in Chapter 12: Skin Tone and Hair Color. The color selection should be close to your natural hair color, as you want to create a natural look. If your natural level is seven, you may select colors from levels five or six, or eight or nine. Refer to Chapter 11: Hairstyling for Your Body Type, Face Shape, and Facial Features for highlighting techniques and placement.

Water/Wood

This is a powerful combination when in balance. Water/Wood types achieve their goals under any circumstances. They are tenacious when they undertake a project. Water people can be reserved until they decide to let their energy shine, while Wood people by nature are gregarious and outgoing—involved in their children's activities and socializing with friends. Water/Wood types love to read. Their appearance reflects the latest fashion. Only when the combination is balanced can their full potential be realized.

The styling for Water element is chic, sensual, flirty, and feminine. The styling for Wood element is active and sporty, with a lot of movement. The challenge is to respect both elements while honoring the dominant one.

Harmonize Water/Wood 2

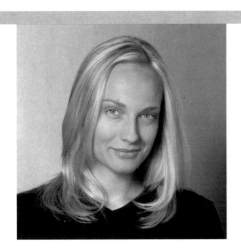

If you measure Yin Extreme or 2 on the Element Barometer, you need to create more control and discipline in your life. I recommend adding Metal to harness the energy of Water. Make a resolution to become organized and on time this year. I know time may not be important to you; however, make your time productive. I recommend adding more structure to your hairstyle in cut and color.

Haircut to Harmonize Water/Wood 2

Harmonize with Metal, adding clean lines while keeping a sensual, active style. Refer to Chapter 11: Hairstyling for Your Body Type, Face Shape, and Facial Features for the best length and cut for you. You want a style with structure and sass.

Hair color to Harmonize Water/Wood 2

Harmonize with Metal by referring to Chapter 12: Skin Tone and Hair Color for color selections according to your skin tone, elements, and natural hair color. If you are a natural level six, you may select from levels three through five, or seven through ten. If you are unsure about a color selection, try a semipermanent color to see if you like it. Refer to Chapter 11: Hairstyling for Your Body Type, Face Shape, and Facial Features for highlighting placement and techniques. Select precise, fine highlights to complement your Metal color.

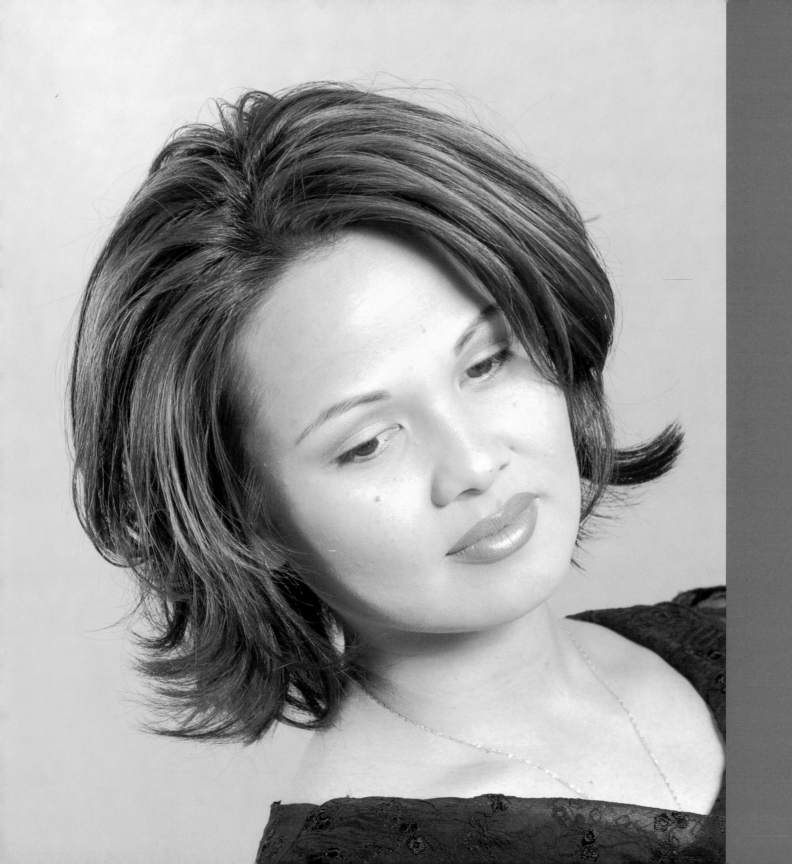

Enhance Water/Wood 4

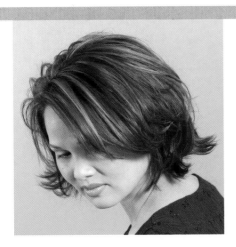

If you measure Yin Moderate or 4 on the Element Barometer, you need to replenish the Water element. Enroll in a yoga class or college night class for self-renewal. I recommend creating a fashion statement with sass.

Haircut to Enhance Water/Wood 4

Enhance with Water, using rounded layers to create a flirty kick. Refer to Chapter 11: Hairstyling for Your Body Type, Face Shape, and Facial Features for the best length and cut. Select a cut that perfectly reflects your sense of who you are.

Hair color to Enhance Water/Wood 4

Enhance with Water by referring to Chapter 12: Skin Tone and Hair Color for color selection based on your skin tone, natural hair color, and elements. If you are a natural level six, you may select colors from levels two through five or seven through eleven. Refer to Chapter 11: Hairstyling for Your Body Type, Face Shape, and Facial Features for highlighting placement and techniques. You want an expressive color and highlights.

Harmonize Water/Wood 6

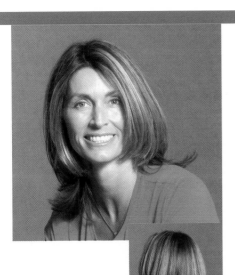

If you measure Yang Moderate or 6 on the Element Barometer, you need to add Wood to diminish the amount of Water in your element. You tend to become isolated and need to become more involved in social activities. I recommend creating movement in your hairstyle.

Haircut to Harmonize Water/Wood 6

Harmonize with Wood, creating texture for movement. The cut can be short, contouring to head shape. If you prefer a longer style, use round layers to keep the ends full, yet flirty, with movement. Refer to Chapter 11: Hairstyling for Your Body Type, Face Shape, and Facial Features for the best cut and style.

Hair color to Harmonize Water/Wood 6

Harmonize with Wood by referring to Chapter 12: Skin Tone and Hair Color for color selections according to your skin tone, element, and natural hair color. If your hair color is a natural level six, you may select from levels four or five, or seven through nine. Refer to Chapter 11: Hairstyling for Your Body Type, Face Shape, and Facial Features for highlighting placement and techniques. I suggest you use both Wood color and Wood highlighting techniques to harmonize.

Balance Water/Wood 8

If you measure Yang Extreme or 8 on the Element Barometer, you need to add Earth to balance the overabundance of Water. I recommend introducing Earth into your life by volunteering to help with a preschool class or to read to an older person who has failing sight. Make a difference in someone's life and you will be amazed by the difference it makes in yours.

Haircut to Balance Water/Wood 8

Balance with Earth by creating soft layers within the cut. Refer to Chapter 11: Hairstyling for Your Body Type, Face Shape, and Facial Features for the best length and cut. You want to create softness with the styling. Remember you don't want to stop up the Water, only slow it down.

Hair color to Balance Water/Wood 8

Balance with Earth by referring to Chapter 12: Skin Tone and Hair Color for color selections based on your skin tone, element, and natural color level. If you are a natural level five, you may select colors from levels three, four, six, or eight. Refer to Chapter 11: Hairstyling for Your Body Type, Face Shape, and Facial Features for highlighting placement and techniques. I would use Earth color and Water highlights to create a soft, natural look. It is important that Water is only tamed, not stopped.

10 Wood Element

Wood types are adventurers. They are outgoing and very social. They are competitive with others and with themselves in achieving their goals. As salespeople, they strive to be number one and will sometimes set impossible goals—they don't like being number two. Wood types are organized and able to focus on any endeavor. They are very likeable and make great friends. A Wood type will know everyone at the party before she leaves. Wood types are active and can multitask with ease. They become successful leaders by being able to compromise without losing integrity. They are the ones to take the ideas of Water types and turn them into reality.

The great outdoors beckons to Wood types and they feel more alive and energetic without the confines of walls. If you need a guide to take you to the most awesome waterfall or to view a hidden cave, Wood types thrive on the journey and will regale you with stories they have gathered in their explorations. Youthful and playful, they bring an infectious energy and enthusiasm to all their activities. If you have a Wood type as a partner or significant other, you will never be bored. Your problem may lie in getting him or her to yourself, as Wood types thrive in a crowd. They are the eternal optimists, even when facing adversity. Even though they are competitive, they also have a kind nature that keeps them from being cutthroat. They will do their best and win if they can, but on ethical terms. Of all the elements, Wood types are the most ethical in relationships. When they are overstressed, they turn to nature for solace. They prefer to be alone while healing and gaining strength for another challenge.

I am fortunate to have a friend who is also a client who epitomizes the Wood type. She seems to be in perpetual motion, yet she never appears to be stressed or rushed. Her calm demeanor belies her active life style. She keeps in shape through daily tennis games and by working out with her personal trainer. Whether it is assisting her husband in their business or volunteering to be the class mom for her three children, she excels in meeting her goals. If one of her friends is in need, she is at the house with food in hand and a ready smile to lift her friend's spirit. Lest you think this lady is a wonder woman, she is an endless fountain of energy who renews her strength by spending time at the ocean alone. Wood types are capable of multitasking and complete each project on time and meet their goals. They are excellent business owners, managers, leaders, and directors. They are great communicators and often select a career that requires communication skills, such as public relations, motivational speaking, television, radio, or mentoring.

Wood types make every event a social event. They love to be around people and seem to draw their energy from the crowd. Not only will they meet most of the people in attendance, but they will remember everyone's name and something about them. That is why they excel as salespeople and leaders of organizations. In some areas, the Wood types are known as those who can work a crowd. Their lack of pretentiousness makes them genuinely liked by most people they encounter. Whenever I attend any function, I am always drawn to the Wood types as they will take time to listen and inquire about your interests. It is not merely nodding the head but a participatory conversation that leaves me feeling exhilarated.

It is the Wood types who keep the spirit of our businesses alive. Whenever we schedule the product of the month contest, we know without a doubt that the contest will be between the Wood types at our different locations. It isn't the prize that serves as the incentive; it is the competition that they relish. Our Wood types serve as the official hosts and hostesses in our salon and spa as they make it a point to speak to each client who enters their area. They are the ones who take the initiative to develop new treatments, services, and ideas for packages or specials. At our salons, we host programs for civic organizations and clubs on Monday evenings. It is the Wood types who will plan the entire event and serve as the host or hostess. If they take on a project, they will see it through to the end. If they are unable to complete the task, they have no difficulty in delegating to someone else. They are definitely people persons.

Wood types' love for adventure and physical activity serves as the basis for their success as athletes. They do equally well competing alone (as in a bicycle race) or when participating as a member of a team. They become almost obsessive about staying in great physical shape, which I believe accounts for their boundless energy. They become involved in finding the best diet that will assist them in staying fit. They are faithful to their workout routines and to their schedules. The key for a Wood type as with all other elements is balance.

Wood types prefer a casual professional look and are not slaves to the latest fashion. They prefer clothes that move with them as they dislike any restrictions in their life or clothing. They must have been the ones who invented "Casual Fridays," as that is their choice of dress. They live an active life and their clothing certainly reflects it. Their hairstyle has to adapt to an active lifestyle during the weekend or after work.

Within each element, Yin and Yang energies exist. On the Element Barometer, I have listed characteristics that will assist you in knowing whether you need to enhance, harmonize, or balance the element. If the Wood element is hidden or Yin Extreme 2, you need to add Water to feed or activate the Wood element. When the Yin is Moderate 4, you need to enhance the Wood by applying more Wood. When the Yang is Moderate 6, you need to add Fire to diminish the Wood's energy. You don't want to burn it down; you want to thin it out so it won't be so dense. When the Yang is Extreme 8, the addition of Metal will give it structure. The amount of Wood we express can be compared to the different types of Wood we use. Desert ironwood is the second-hardest wood and is used for support. That is similar to a Yang Extreme Wood 8 on the Element Barometer. A Yang Moderate Wood 6 is similar to mahogany that is used for building fine tables or dressers. A Yin Moderate Wood 4 is much like hickory in that it is strong but bendable. A Yin Extreme Wood 2 is like white pine—a soft, pliable wood that is used to make inexpensive furniture.

Using Feng Shui principles designed to bring balance and create a flow of good Chi, I take into consideration not only your haircut, hair color, makeup, body type, and face shape, but also your hobbies, lifestyle, exercise patterns, meditation habits, clothing, and accessories. All of these things affect you and the image you portray. When I prescribe the look that will best affect how you perceive yourself, I also address other factors that influence your life. Some of the changes or recommendations will be evident almost immediately such as haircut, hair color, and makeup. The other changes require more of your participation and will evolve, as you are the one in charge of implementing that part of your life. The amount of change will depend upon your dedication.

Makeup for the Wood Element

Soft, natural arrays of color are recommended for the Wood types. Wood techniques are basic and rely on your natural beauty. You don't want to hide or cover up; you want to enhance and protect. Use makeup to enhance your best features. Keep your lips lubricated when participating in activities—you can use gloss over color for your lips. Sun damage is the primary cause of premature aging, so protect your skin while you are outdoors, always wear sunscreen, and limit your time in the midday sun.

Porcelain
Try a soft shimmer of pink dusted across eyelids with pink to nude gloss on lips.

Milky
Use ivory and brown eye shadow with nude to peach lip gloss.

Honey
Apply shades of brown eye shadow, with peach to brownish on the lips.

Olive
Apply a light touch of berry to eyelids, with mauve to pink gloss on lips.

Ebony
Try oranges, reds, and browns on eyes and lips.

Ruby
Use bone, nude, or brown on eyes, and nude on the lips.

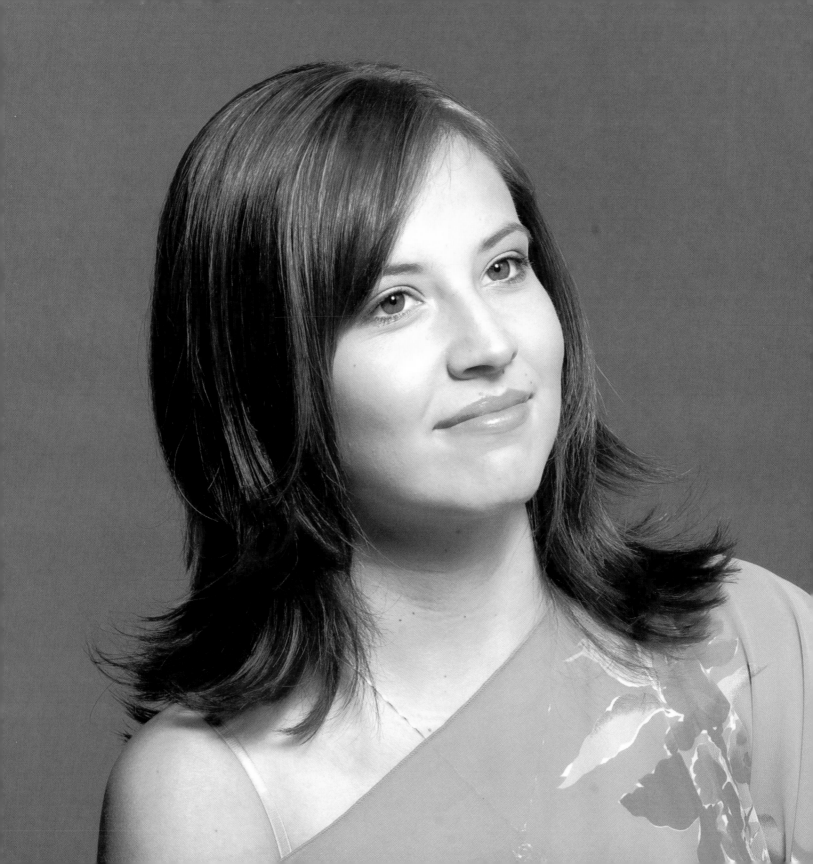

Wood/Fire

Wood/Fire types are the ones who fidget in meetings and in school. They learn quickly and become bored just sitting. This is a very exciting combination. They are very social and make friends easily. They are the types that have never met a stranger. However, they also lose interest quickly. They are the jack of all trades and sports. They will try a new sport, conquer it, and then move on to another one. Since Wood feeds Fire, it is a very volatile combination. It is important to keep these types balanced.

One of my employees decided to join a gym as a social activity (in other words, to meet guys). She had been active in sports while in high school, but she had gotten lackadaisical while going to beauty school and starting her career. A client of hers invited her to try her gym, and she began to meet her friend there every evening after work. Soon she had so much energy that her excitement influenced some of her younger coworkers to join her at the gym. As her body became fit, she became almost obsessed with achieving more. She was in competition with herself. Her work became more creative and she became one of our busiest stylists within a few years. She also achieved her original goal, meeting a man—who became her husband—at the gym! She is truly a Wood/Fire balance.

Harmonize Wood/Fire 2

If you measure Yin Extreme or 2 on the Element Barometer, you need to add Water to bring out the best in Wood. Be careful and don't add too much as it will overwhelm Wood. I suggest that you select a favorite book or go to a concert in the park during your leisure time. I recommend adding a Water cut, color, or highlights, but not all three at once.

Haircut to Harmonize Wood/Fire 2

Harmonize with Water by creating flirty, textured ends on the style for pizzazz. Refer to Chapter 11: Hairstyling for Your Body Type, Face Shape, and Facial Features for the best length and cut. If you have curly hair, I recommend styling the hair into spiraling curls for a sensual style. Cut into curly hair to create volume and separation.

Hair color to Harmonize Wood/Fire 2

Colors should be vibrant and alive. Harmonize with Water by referring to Chapter 12: Skin Tone and Hair Color for color selection based on your skin tone, element, and natural hair level. If you are a natural level six, you may select colors from levels two through five or seven through eleven. Refer to Chapter 11: Hairstyling for Your Body Type, Face Shape, and Facial Features for highlighting placement and techniques.

Enhance Wood/Fire 4

If you measure Yin Moderate or 4 on the Element Barometer, you need to strengthen your Wood element. Take the opportunity to get in shape again by scheduling a power walk with a friend or joining a gym. Maybe kayaking or mountain climbing are more your style. You need fresh air to be healthy and outdoor activities are perfect for you to build strength. In beauty, I recommend adding movement in your cut and color.

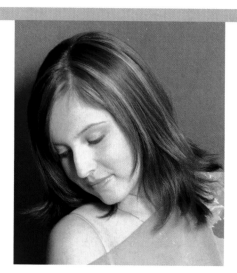

Haircut to Enhance Wood/Fire 4

Enhance with Wood by adding long layers that are textured for support and movement, creating a sexy style. If you prefer your hair shorter, select a cut that has texture at the ends. You want a style that looks great without requiring a lot of styling product. Refer to Chapter 11: Hairstyling for Your Body Type, Face Shape, and Facial Features for the best length and cut for you.

Hair color to Enhance Wood/Fire 4

Enhance with Wood colors as listed in Chapter 12: Skin Tone and Hair Color. The selection of colors is based on your skin tone, elements, and natural hair level. If you are a natural level five, you may select colors from levels three or four, or six through eight. Refer to Chapter 11: Hairstyling for Your Body Type, Face Shape, and Facial Features for highlighting placement and techniques. You can be expressive and creative with the highlights.

Harmonize Wood/Fire 6

If you measure Yang Moderate or 6 on the Element Barometer, you need to add Fire. A little Fire will cause the Wood to stop and focus. It will also encourage more passion about life and less need to be so transient. Follow your dreams and spend a week in New York seeing all of the hit plays on Broadway, or travel to Paris for lunch at a sidewalk café. If travel is out of the question, you could try writing, painting, or dancing to express your creativity.

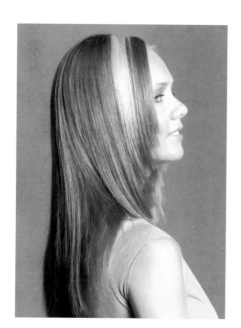

Haircut to Harmonize Wood/Fire 6

Harmonize with Fire to create a disconnected, channel cut while keeping texture for support. You want a bold look without chaos. Refer to Chapter 11: Hairstyling for Your Body Type, Face Shape, and Facial Features for the best length and haircut. Be willing to try a new style. If you have thin or fine hair, you might prefer an asymmetrical hairstyle or one reminiscent of the art of Pablo Picasso. This style would also work if you have curly hair.

Hair color to Harmonize Wood/Fire 6

Harmonize with Fire by referring to Chapter 12: Skin Tone and Hair Color for color selections based on your natural level, skin tone, and element. Any color will work for Fire elements as long as it matches their skin tone. You are the one who decides how daring you want to be. Refer to Chapter 11: Hairstyling for Your Body Type, Face Shape, and Facial Features for highlighting techniques and placement. I would recommend selecting either Fire highlights or Fire color at first. If you select both with a Fire haircut, it may be too much too soon. You may not want a drastic makeover at first; take it in two steps so you'll be comfortable.

Balance Wood/Fire 8

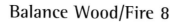

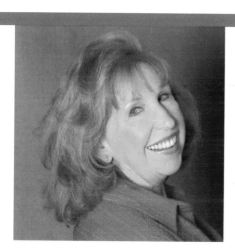

If you measure 8 on the Element Barometer, you need to add Metal to balance. Metal brings order and boundaries when our lives appear out of control. Metal can chop, prune, or conquer Wood depending on how much you add. I recommend adding only one service of Metal. Look at your life and see what needs to be more structured. You can begin by organizing your day, your car, your closet, or your home. You decide what will assist you to become more disciplined. In beauty I look for a sleek, precise style instead of one free-flowing with movement.

Haircut to Balance Wood/Fire 8

Balance with Metal techniques, using clean lines that kick at the ends. You are slowing the movement but not stopping it. Turn to Chapter 11 to select your best length and cut. The cut will not be a precision cut, but rather a cut that is more textured at the ends.

Hair color to Balance Wood/Fire 8

Balance with Metal by referring to Chapter 12: Skin Tone and Hair Color for color selections according to your skin tone, element, and natural hair color. If you are a natural level six, you may select color from levels three through five, or seven through ten. Refer to Chapter 11: Hairstyling for Your Body Type, Face Shape, and Facial Features for highlighting techniques and placement. If you select Metal highlighting techniques, you will have very fine and precise highlights.

Wood/Earth

Everyone should be so lucky as to have this combination for a friend, coworker, or partner. They are easygoing and patient. Wood is friendly and outgoing, while Earth is very nurturing, so the result is a friendly, caring individual. Wood types tend to lose interest quickly, while Earth likes stability and repetition. Wood/Earth needs to be in balance to reap the best of both elements.

I am blessed to have a client that is the nursing supervisor of a large hospital in Los Angeles. Most of her work is on the management level now; however, she has over twenty years of experience in nursing in all departments. She is well respected in the industry and by her coworkers. She has risen to the top of her profession and now has enrolled for more advanced training so she can teach at the university level. Although she has been offered numerous opportunities for positions outside the nursing and medical field, she has chosen to stay true to her love for caring and sharing with others.

After work, she returns home to her three children and husband. She and her husband are involved in activities with their children. She is a fanatic about walking on her treadmill before work and working out at the gym on her days off and whenever she can manage any spare time. Her backyard serves as a magnet for all of her neighbors as the meeting place. Whether it is a Fourth of July cookout, someone's birthday, or just a great day to socialize, a party invitation will arrive by a phone call. She can balance both her elements better than most I have observed.

Harmonize Wood/Earth 2

If you measure Yin Extreme or 2 on the Element Barometer, you need to add Water to add more chic to your style. Water is more fashion-conscious that either Wood or Earth. Spend a day browsing through magazines or through the mall (leave your money at home so you won't be tempted). You want to see the latest styles and be aware of how you can incorporate the looks you like with what's in.

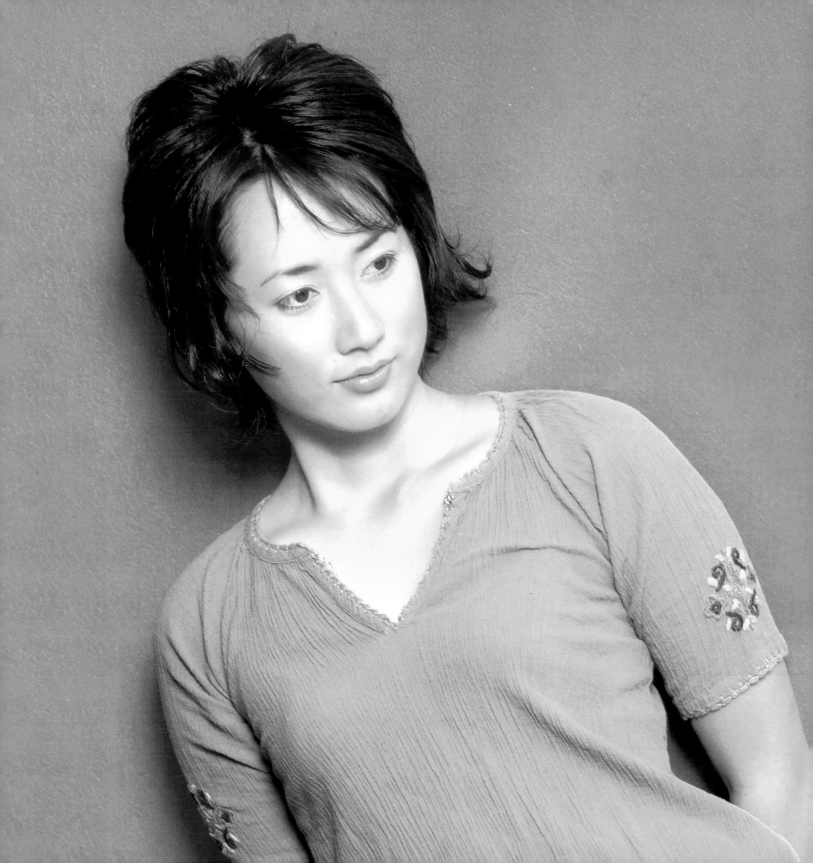

Haircut to Harmonize Wood/Earth 2

Harmonize with Water, adding round layers to give a sporty, flirty look. The key to the style is texturizing the ends. Refer to Chapter 11: Hairstyling for Your Body Type, Face Shape, and Facial Features for the best length and cut. I recommend blending the chic of Water with the sporty look of Wood.

Hair color to Harmonize Wood/Earth 2

Harmonize with Water colors by referring to Chapter 12: Skin Tone and Hair Color for hair color selection based on your skin tone, natural hair color, and element. If you are a natural level five, you may select colors from levels one through four, or six through ten. You have a wider range of colors available with Water than with Wood or Earth. Wood and Earth require that you select colors closer to your natural level. Refer to Chapter 11: Hairstyling for Your Body Type, Face Shape, and Facial Features for highlighting techniques and placement.

Enhance Wood/Earth 4

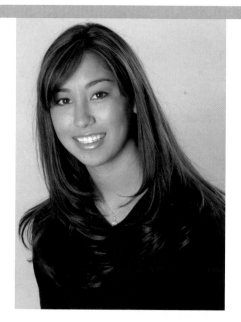

If you measure Yin Moderate or 4 on the Element Barometer, your Wood needs strengthening. It is necessary to add Wood to bring out the optimism and the brilliance you have hidden. Add more Wood element to your life by taking a public speaking course at your local college, enrolling in a gym, or joining a swim team. If those activities are not to your liking, I suggest finding one that not only involves others but that will require physical activity. In your appearance, I would look for a more natural hairstyle and hair color.

Haircut to Enhance Wood/Earth 4

Enhance with Wood, creating natural lines with movement—a clean, no-fuss style. Wood haircuts have swing or movement within the haircut and at the ends. You want a look that is easy to maintain, but that will work for you in your career. On the weekend or during your leisure time, you will want a style that doesn't require a lot of styling products to look good. Refer to Chapter 11: Hairstyling for Your Body Type, Face Shape, and Facial Features for the best length and cut for you.

Hair color to Enhance Wood/Earth 4

Enhance with Wood by referring to Chapter 12: Skin Tone and Hair Color for color selection based on your natural hair color, skin tone, and element. If you are a natural level five, you may select colors from levels three or four, or six through eight. You will want to change the depth of your color according to the seasons. In the summer months, your skin tone may change depending on the amount of time you stay in the sun. Refer to Chapter 11: Hairstyling for Your Body Type, Face Shape, and Facial Features for highlighting techniques and placement.

Harmonize Wood/Earth 6

If you measure Yang Moderate or 6 on the Element Barometer, you need to add Fire for a more fun and free style. You want to decrease the Wood that always needs to be on the go and socially involved. Fire element will inspire Wood element to find a creative outlet. Fire will allow your hidden passion to become central to your decision making. In beauty, I recommend an expressive look that throws caution to the wind.

Haircut to Harmonize Wood/Earth 6

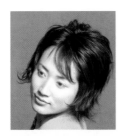

Harmonize with Fire, using softer pieces to create a more artistic edge. I would not create a bold, disconnected style—just enough texture to be expressive. It is up to you to determine how creative you want your hairstyle to be. Refer to Chapter 11: Hairstyling for Your Body Type, Face Shape, and Facial Features for the best length and haircut. If you prefer your hair longer, make certain that it has enough texture for a wild, wind-blown look. Have fun with your new look.

Hair color to Harmonize Wood/Earth 6

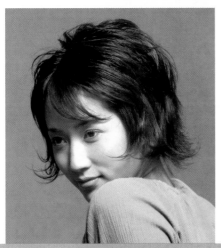

Harmonize with Fire by referring to Chapter 12: Skin Tone and Hair Color for color selection according to your skin tone, natural hair level, and element. It doesn't matter what your natural color level is; you may select any color as long as it matches your skin tone. If your skin is porcelain, which is a cool tone, you would select your colors from the cool tones in your hair color choices. Refer to Chapter 11: Hairstyling for Your Body Type, Face Shape, and Facial Features for highlighting techniques and placement. I would not use both Fire highlighting techniques and Fire colors. Try using Wood color and Fire highlighting techniques, or vice versa.

Balance Wood/Earth 8

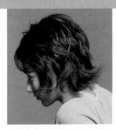

If you measure Yang Extreme or 8 on the Element Barometer, you need to add Metal to balance your Wood element. Sometimes Wood types are too spontaneous and aggressive. They need to have discipline and focus in order to be balanced and reach Wood's maximum potential. Take up chess or challenge yourself with crossword puzzles. Clean your closet and neatly store items that don't fit. If clothing has not been worn in two years, donate it to a charity or homeless center or stage a garage sale. For your hairstyle, I recommend a classic look rather than a tousled, windblown style.

Haircut to Balance Wood/Earth 8

Balance with Metal, creating a stylish, fashionable cut with soft, classic lines. Feel free to choose a classic bob and have it softened for your Wood/Earth taste. Refer to Chapter 11: Hairstyling for Your Body Type, Face Shape, and Facial Features for the best length and haircut. If you are feeling organized and want your look to reflect this trait, then go for a total Metal cut that is sharp, sleek, and classically elegant.

Hair color to Balance Wood/Earth 8

Balance with Metal by referring to Chapter 12: Skin Tone and Hair Color for color selections according to your skin tone, element, and natural hair color. Metal element offers a wider selection of colors than Wood or Earth. If you are a natural level five, you may select colors from levels two through four or six through nine. Refer to Chapter 11: Hairstyling for Your Body Type, Face Shape, and Facial Features for highlighting techniques and placement. Choosing both Metal colors and Metal techniques may be too restrictive for a social Wood/Earth. You decide how much change you want and do it either gradually or all at once. Enjoy your choices.

Wood/Metal

Wood/Metal types are very steadfast and loyal. They can also be very charming, but usually not in a large crowd. The Metal element furnishes the discipline and focus that may be missing for Wood element types. When in balance, Wood/Metal types prove to be excellent business leaders. They have the winning combination of being social, competitive, and organized. They can withstand pressure and stay true to their values. They are very tenacious about achieving their goals, and on time. Wood/Metal types never mind delegating and following up to see that the project is completed to their standards. They may need the extra thanks or a pat on the shoulder for a job well done. Often, they are so efficient that others take them for granted. They are great at negotiating in business and winning the trust of those they encounter. Integrity is

extremely important to them. They are loyal to the few friends they include in their inner circle.

A close business associate of mine is a Wood/Metal and prides herself in completing her tasks on time and being at the top in her company. She is as comfortable hosting a large gathering as communicating one-on-one. Her Metal influence keeps her on track and she is able to accomplish a great deal in a short period of time. She competes with herself to best her last year's income and productivity. This competitive characteristic comes through when she urges her children to excel and to reach for their dreams. She stays in physical shape by walking on her treadmill and following an exercise routine designed by her personal trainer. Her hairstyle is Wood harmonized with Fire, her clothing style is a combination of Metal and Wood, and her makeup is Wood. She makes a striking impression in her appearance and in her demeanor.

Harmonize Wood/Metal 2

If you measure Yin Extreme or 2 on the Element Barometer, your Wood element is hidden and needs the addition of Water element. Water will enhance the growth of Wood and will give Wood more expression. Water types are thoughtful and look to the future for their growth. When Wood types are not expressed, they become too scattered and lose their strength. I recommend that Wood types read and listen to speakers on spirituality and self-growth. In your hairstyle, I recommend a sensual, chic look.

Haircut to Harmonize Wood/Metal 2

Harmonize with Water using classic lines, breaking up to make it more chic, yet active. This cut will honor your Wood element with an active touch, your Metal element with the classic lines, and your Water element with a chic look, bringing you in balance for good Chi. Refer to Chapter 11: Hairstyling for Your Body Type, Face Shape, and Facial Features for your best length and haircut. You decide if you want a complete makeover or want to create your new look gradually.

Hair color to Harmonize Wood/Metal 2

Harmonize with Water element by referring to Chapter 12: Skin Tone and Hair Color for color selection according to your skin tone, element, and natural hair color. If you are a natural level six, you may select colors from levels two through five or seven through eleven. That is a wide range of colors; make certain that you pay attention to your skin tone when selecting your color. Refer to Chapter 11: Hairstyling for Your Body Type, Face Shape, and Facial Features for highlighting techniques and placement. I would recommend using both Water color and Water highlighting techniques. This combination needs the pizzazz.

Enhance Wood/Metal 4

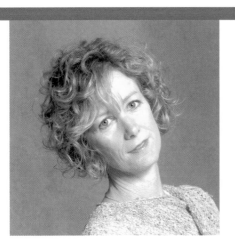

If you measure Yin Moderate or 4, you need to increase your Wood element. Add more activities to your life—turn off the television and get involved in an organization or club that requires you to become more social. Take classes in leadership or utilize the abilities that lie dormant. I recommend adding Wood to your cut and your color.

Haircut to Enhance Wood/Metal 4

Enhance with Wood, creating natural lines with movement for a clean, no-fuss style. You want to honor your secondary element as well as enhance your dominant one. Select a style that is free-flowing with natural lines and still looks professional. Refer to Chapter 11: Hairstyling for Your Body Type, Face Shape, and Facial Features for the best length and cut.

Hair color to Enhance Wood/Metal 4

Enhance with Wood by referring to Chapter 12: Skin Tone and Hair Color for color selection according to your skin tone, natural hair color, and element. If you are a natural level five, you may select colors from levels three or four, or six through eight. Refer to Chapter 11: Hairstyling for Your Body Type, Face Shape, and Facial Features for highlighting techniques and placement. I recommend using both Wood color and Wood highlighting techniques.

Harmonize Wood/Metal 6

If you measure Yang Moderate or 6 on the Element Barometer, harmonize with Fire to create more expression and to control the Wood. Attend a concert in the park or attend a great movie. Go for the pleasure and for the fun. Buy an article of clothing that is colorful and trendy. Change the dials on your radio and listen to a different genre of music. Check out the latest art showing at your favorite gallery. Get some fun and laughter back into your life to lift your spirits and build your immune system. For fashion, I want to see a "Wow!" effect when you walk into a room. This may take time to achieve, as your secondary element is reserved.

Haircut to Harmonize Wood/Metal 6

Harmonize with Fire, using uneven texture for movement within the haircut. Select a cut that you never thought was for you. Begin gradually with the cut suggested above and, as you feel more expressive, you can go as bold as you like. Refer to Chapter 11: Hairstyling for Your Body Type, Face Shape, and Facial Features for the best length and haircut. You want a creative and expressive cut.

Hair color to Harmonize Wood/Metal 6

Harmonize with Fire by referring to Chapter 12: Skin Tone and Hair Color for color selection according to your skin tone, element, and natural hair color. You are lucky, as the only limits for a Fire element is skin tone. You might want to start with a level very close to your natural level. You be the judge. Refer to Chapter 11: Hairstyling for Your Body Type, Face Shape, and Facial Features for highlighting techniques and placement. I recommend that you use Fire for either color or highlighting, and Wood for the other.

Balance Wood/Metal 8

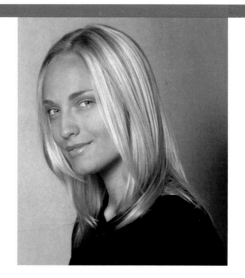

If you measure Yang Extreme or 8 on the Element Barometer, you need to add Metal to diminish the effects of too much Wood. Metal will add structure and discipline to Wood. Enroll in a college class or attend a Shakespeare reading or play. Read the classics again (or for the first time). Buy a book on crossword puzzles or engage in a game of Scrabble. You want to become focused on achieving your goals. In fashion, you want to slow down the movement with classic lines and colors.

Haircut to Balance Wood/Metal 8

Balance with Metal to create a classic, refined style that is sophisticated, yet sporty. It sounds like a contradiction, but it will give you a progressive, classic look. Think of a classic bob that you can tuck behind your ears for a more casual look. You don't want a look that boxes you in. Refer to Chapter 11: Hairstyling for Your Body Type, Face Shape, and Facial Features for the best length and haircut for you.

Hair color to Balance Wood/Metal 8

Balance with Metal by referring to Chapter 12: Skin Tone and Hair Color for color selection according to your skin tone, natural hair color, and element. If you are a natural level five, you may select colors from levels two through four, or six through nine. Refer to Chapter 11: Hairstyling for Your Body Type, Face Shape, and Facial Features for highlighting techniques and placement. Metal highlighting techniques are precise and refined. If you select Metal colors, I recommend you use Metal highlighting techniques.

Wood/Water

Wood/Water types have the characteristics to be the best: Wood type is social, seeking advancement, while Water type is the thinker or visionary who can seal success. The challenge occurs when obstacles come their way; they tend to get bogged down with excuses. Left to themselves, they find a way to balance any setbacks and don't need others to boost their self image. If you have a Wood/Water for a friend, be sure to lend a shoulder when they become emotionally drained—and they will.

A business associate of mine is a Wood/Water type. His social life consists of parties—when it is advantageous for his business—or nights at home reading, researching the latest technology and finding ways to incorporate it into his business. His work consists of creating virtual reality shows for large corporations to showcase their businesses. He went to one of my platform presentations and was waiting for me backstage as soon as my performance ended. He said, "Why just tell them the characteristics of Fire? I can have a flash of Fire envelope the room using virtual reality. Water becomes more than words, it becomes a wave of Water to show the intensity according to the level of Water in your life." I have since visited his business, where he has a theater for showcasing his proposals for his clients. He has to be a visionary, as that is what he sells, and he has to be social and outgoing in order to be competitive. His shelves of awards attest to his success.

Harmonize Wood/Water 2

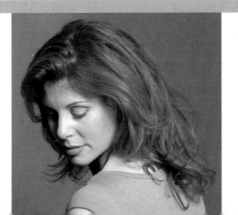

If you measure Yin Extreme or 2 on the Element Barometer, introduce the Water element for more vitality and flexibility. Water feeds Wood and spurs its growth. Read autobiographies and books about new ideas for inspiration. I recommend honoring the Water element by creating a chic, flirty look to your appearance.

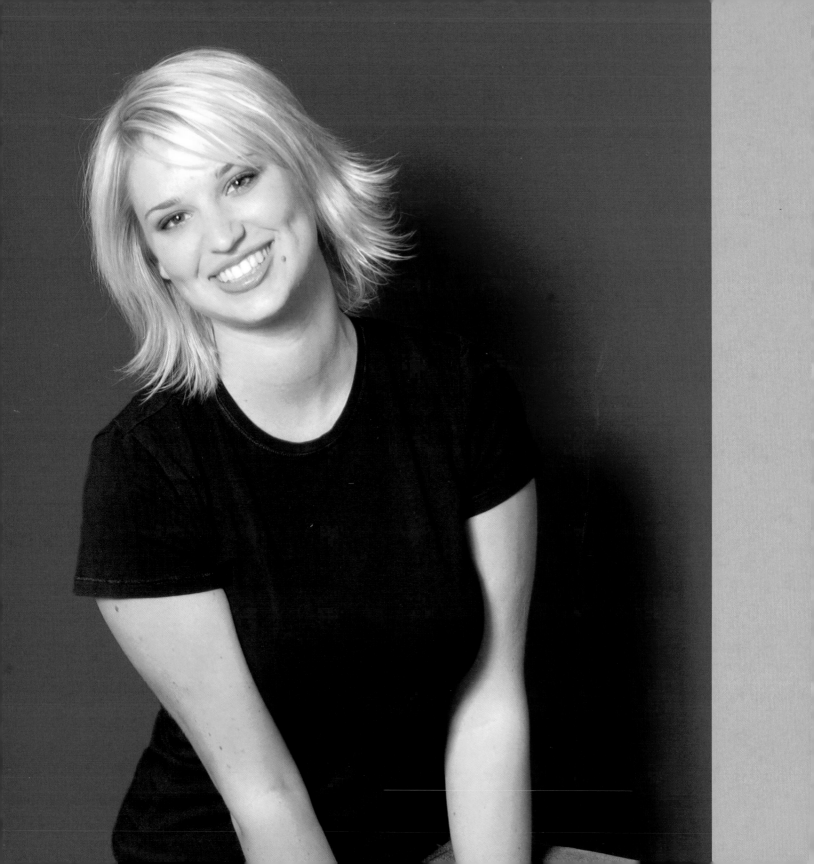

Haircut to Harmonize Wood/Water 2

Harmonize with Water, using texture in the haircut to create a sensual attitude. You want to avoid the windblown effect and achieve a look that says there is more here than meets the eye. Make them lean forward to hear what you have to say—and then have something to say. Refer to Chapter 11: Hairstyling for Your Body Type, Face Shape, and Facial Features for the best length and cut.

Hair color to Harmonize Wood/Water 2

Harmonize with Water by referring to Chapter 12: Skin Tone and Hair Color for color selection based on your skin tone, natural hair color level, and element. Refer to Chapter 11: Hairstyling for Your Body Type, Face Shape, and Facial Features for highlighting techniques and placement. I recommend using both Water highlighting techniques and Water color selections.

Enhance Wood/Water 4

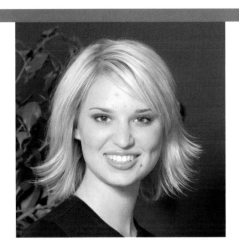

If you measure Yin Moderate or 4 on the Element Barometer, you need to express more Wood. Become active again in your sports of choice. It is good to be a fan, but also become actively involved in a physical activity for increased energy. Plan a party for friends or relatives. You love being around others, and when your Wood element is feeling weak, you need to spur its growth by socializing more.

Haircut to Enhance Wood/Water 4

Enhance with Wood by adding long, rounded layers that sway in or out with head movement. If you select a short- or medium-length haircut, you can still get rounded layers. Refer to Chapter 11: Hairstyling for Your Body Type, Face Shape, and Facial Features for your best length and haircut. You want a look that moves and is ready to go when you are.

Hair color to Enhance Wood/Water 4

Enhance with Wood by referring to Chapter 12: Skin Tone and Hair Color for color selection according to your skin tone, element, and natural hair color. If you are a level seven, you may select colors from levels five or six, or eight through ten. Refer to Chapter 11: Hairstyling for Your Body Type, Face Shape, and Facial Features for highlighting techniques and placement. I would use both Wood color and Wood highlighting techniques.

Harmonize Wood/Water 6

If you measure Yang Moderate or 6 on the Element Barometer, add Fire to slow down Wood and keep it from growing so rapidly. Too much Fire can destroy Wood, but the right amount can keep Wood vital. Dig out your old paintbrushes and begin your masterpiece—just for you. Rediscover your passion in life and follow your dreams. Find a way to express the artistic side of you, whether in storytelling, writing, entertaining, or in your clothing. When you create, you become more open to new ideas which represent growth. Have fun creating and release your inhibitions, at least for a little while. In fashion, I am looking for color and expression.

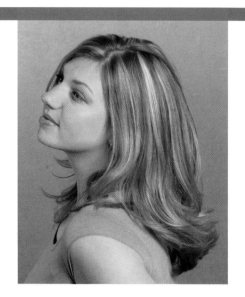

Haircut to Harmonize Wood/Water 6

Harmonize with Fire, keeping the style textured with sexy pieces in the length. You can be as expressive as you dare. Try a new cut that is edgy but that also permits you to style it in a professional manner for your work. Use products to create that textured look when you desire. Refer to Chapter 11: Hairstyling for Your Body Type, Face Shape, and Facial Features for the best length and cut.

Hair color to Harmonize Wood/Water 6

Harmonize with Fire by referring to Chapter 12: Skin Tone and Hair Color for color selection based on your skin tone, natural hair color, and element. With Fire element, your color selection is limited only by your skin tone and your imagination. Refer to Chapter 11: Hairstyling for Your Body Type, Face Shape, and Facial Features for highlighting techniques and placement. I would use Fire color as well as Fire techniques for an expressive style.

Balance Wood/Water 8

If you measure Yang Extreme or 8 on the Element Barometer, add Metal to balance and control the Wood. Find a hobby that intrigues you and challenges your intellect. Metal types thrive on organized surroundings, from their closet to their cars. Make certain that you clean the clutter from your environment as well as from your life. An organized mind can complete tasks more quickly and efficiently. For your appearance, I prefer a structured look that has a sense of movement.

Haircut to Balance Wood/Water 8

Balance with Metal by cutting in a classic style, while keeping texture at the ends. You want your hair to look controlled and professional, rather than casual. Think of a precision cut that suggests movement. Refer to Chapter 11: Hairstyling for Your Body Type, Face Shape, and Facial Features for the best length and cut.

Hair color to Balance Wood/Water 8

Balance with Metal by referring to Chapter 12: Skin Tone and Hair Color for color selection based on your skin tone, natural hair color, and element. If you are a natural level six, you may select colors from levels three through five or seven through ten. Refer to Chapter 11: Hairstyling for Your Body Type, Face Shape, and Facial Features for highlighting techniques and placement. I would use either Metal highlighting techniques or Metal color, but not both, as the result would be too refined for Wood/Water.

Wood/Wood

A whirlwind of energy describes the Wood/Wood types. They are always on the go, seeking new opportunities, traveling, trying new jobs, or moving to new houses. Wood types love to learn and take classes throughout their life, always wanting to better themselves. They tend to imagine the worst case scenario. They have great imaginations and can spin a story or create an exciting event out of the most mundane happening. If you have friends who are Wood/Wood types, they can drain you with their energy or boost you when you need it the most. They are willing to try anything once, even if odds are that it will fail. There's always the possibility that it won't, and they will learn something useful along the way. Every experience is exciting.

Wood/Wood types volunteer for their company softball team, plan the annual company party, and introduce the newest employee to the rest of the team. Wood/Wood types serve as official greeters, whether the party is at their home or they are invited guests. Whenever I am around a Wood/Wood type for a prolonged period, I am left either breathless or energized, depending on whether the Wood/Wood type is balanced. They seem to have an innate desire to be liked by all. They don't brood if it doesn't happen, but it does bother them. When they need to slow down, they will find an outdoor setting to replenish their energy. When they return, they will regale you with stories of their experiences.

Their sense of style requires fashion that moves and is unrestricted. They project the image of being "always on the go," and they are never happier than when they really are on the go. They know every team in a national league and

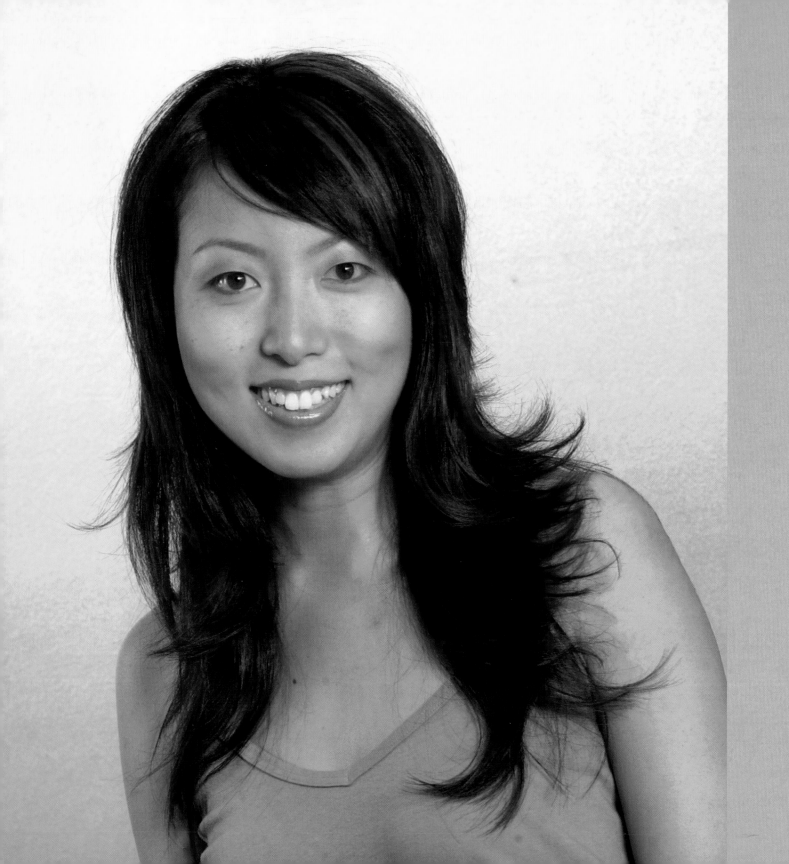

can readily give you stats on the best players. If you need someone to accompany you to the races or ball game, call your Wood/Wood friend. Everyone needs a Wood/Wood type in his/her life.

Harmonize Wood/Wood 2

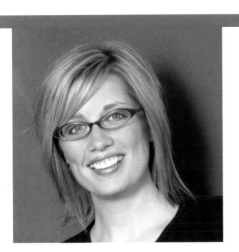

If you measure Yin Extreme or 2 on the Element Barometer, introduce Water to create more energy and feed Wood's growth. Water types serve as visionaries in businesses and in families. What stirs your curiosity about the future? What will next year's styles be? How can you expand your business to be on the cutting edge? If this doesn't interest you, find a book that will allow you to grow spiritually as well as emotionally. Water types have a love for knowledge and are able to utilize this knowledge to create a better world. They are great motivators and educators. In fashion, Water types are sophisticated, and are confident sharing their sensual side.

Haircut to Harmonize Wood/Wood 2

Harmonize with Water by creating a tousled style with a flirty, chic, kicky movement. You want a look that turns heads and makes people listen to you. Refer to Chapter 11: Hairstyling for Your Body Type, Face Shape, and Facial Features for the best length and cut. Have fun with this haircut, as it should be very expressive.

Hair color to Harmonize Wood/Wood 2

Harmonize with Water by referring to Chapter 12: Skin Tone and Hair Color for color selection based on your skin tone, natural hair color, and element. If you are a natural level six, you may select colors from levels two through five or seven through eleven. The Water element has a wide range of colors available. Select one that makes you most comfortable; after all, this is about balancing your Chi. Refer to Chapter 11: Hairstyling for Your Body Type, Face Shape, and Facial Features for highlighting techniques and placement. I recommend using both Water color and Water highlighting techniques.

Enhance Wood/Wood 4

If you measure Yin Moderate or 4 on the Element Barometer, add more Wood to enhance. Add Wood sparingly, as too much can be damaging. Get active, whether it is gardening at home, practicing yoga with a friend, or walking on the treadmill every morning. Activity increases your energy, which increases your Wood element. You need to stay involved. You decide how involved you want to be with outside organizations and learn to set limits so your Wood isn't depleted. I recommend a style for your active life that is free flowing, flattering, and easy to maintain.

Haircut to Enhance Wood/Wood 4
Enhance with Wood by creating a tousled, sporty, bouncy style with soft movement within the haircut. Refer to Chapter 11: Hairstyling for Your Body Type, Face Shape, and Facial Features for your best length and cut. Select a style that will move with you and that reflects who you are.

Hair color to Enhance Wood/Wood 4
Enhance with Wood by referring to Chapter 12: Skin Tone and Hair Color for color selection based on your skin tone, natural hair color, and element. If you are a natural level six, you may select colors from levels four or five, or seven through nine. Refer to Chapter 11: Hairstyling for Your Body Type, Face Shape, and Facial Features for highlighting techniques and placement. I recommend using both Wood colors and Wood highlighting techniques.

Harmonize Wood/Wood 6

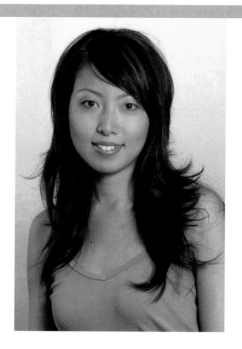

If you measure Yang Moderate or 6 on the Element Barometer, add Fire to help free the Wood from being too harsh. Have fun with the introduction of Fire element in your lifestyle and your appearance. Remember the dreams that you put aside when you grew up? This is the time to revisit your passions and regain that youthful glow. You decide how and when you want to spark that passion in your life. For me, I have a passion for the beauty industry and my choice of career. That is why I feel that when you enjoy what you do, you never go to work. You spend your days fulfilling your dream. In fashion, look for excitement and a dramatic style.

Haircut to Harmonize Wood/Wood 6
Harmonize with Fire, using texture to create an edgier style with movement within the haircut. You decide how creative you want your haircut to be. I recommend that you take sacred steps toward achieving your makeover. I believe it has to come from inside, as well as from your appearance. Refer to Chapter 11: Hairstyling for Your Body Type, Face Shape, and Facial Features for your best length and cut.

Hair color to Harmonize Wood/Wood 6

Harmonize with Fire by referring to Chapter 12: Skin Tone and Hair Color for color selection based on your skin tone, natural hair color, and element. Your only limitations are your skin tone—and your willingness for a complete makeover. Refer to Chapter 11: Hairstyling for Your Body Type, Face Shape, and Facial Features for highlighting techniques and placement. I recommend using either Fire color or Fire highlighting techniques, but not both.

Balance Wood/Wood 8

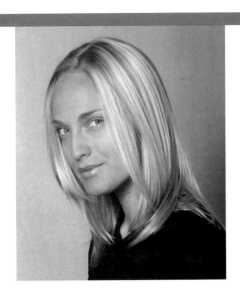

If you measure Yang Extreme or 8 on the Element Barometer, add Metal for the focus to balance scattered Wood. Find an area in your life that needs to be organized or changed. Metal elements have the discipline to achieve their goals. That discipline is vital in organizing your life for success. You are the one that takes inventory of your life and determines how to correct the areas that need to be changed. I recommend a structured look that is not too sharp and confined.

Haircut to Balance Wood/Wood 8

Balance with Metal by using softer, flowing classic lines in the cut. You want structure, not restriction, in the movement of the hair. Refer to Chapter 11: Hairstyling for Your Body Type, Face Shape, and Facial Features for the best length and cut. You may want to add a classic edge to your haircut gradually. The decision is yours.

Hair color to Balance Wood/Wood 8

Balance with Metal by referring to Chapter 12: Skin Tone and Hair Color for color selection based on your skin tone, natural hair color, and element. If you are a natural level six, you may select colors from levels three through five or seven through ten. Refer to Chapter 11: Hairstyling for Your Body Type, Face Shape, and Facial Features for highlighting techniques and placement. I recommend starting with both Metal color and highlights for a beautiful, precise complement to your skin tone and element.

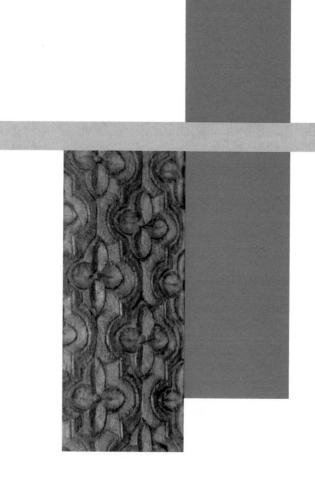

11 Hairstyling

for Your Body Type, Face Shape, and Facial Features

My training in beauty school was as a conventional hairstylist. I learned the usual information: about hair textures, a small amount about face shapes and facial features, and the standard haircuts that were required to pass the state board test to receive my license. After several years of training within a salon, I learned to categorize my clients according to their lifestyle and to cut their hair the way I thought would match that lifestyle. Although I had a great client base and my schedule was full, I wasn't fully satisfied with my career. I felt that something was missing, as my consultation dealt only with my observations.

I have had the good fortune to study with masters in the hair industry: Vidal Sassoon, who revolutionized the beauty industry by creating the techniques for precision cutting, and Horst Rechelbacher of Aveda, who revolutionized the beauty product industry by introducing awareness of aromatherapy and our environment. But the work wasn't done yet. A mentor of mine, Horst said to me, "Billy, complete the triangle." I began to look for a method of helping my clients become a more integral participant in their consultation. This dialogue provided me with more information that influenced their image and desired look. When I incorporated Feng Shui into our salon, everything began to click into place. Everything that I have learned as a stylist serves as a foundation for Feng Shui beauty.

Most people have seen great haircuts in magazines, on celebrities, on friends, or on television, and have taken the pictures or described them to their hair stylist. My clients come into the salon dying to have the latest, most beautiful cut. When Meg Ryan changes her hairstyle, women flock to the salons wanting the same cut and color. The same thing happened when Jennifer Aniston had the "Rachel" cut. Everyone wanted it. It is rare when anyone stops to think about the factors that go into making the haircut the perfect cut for the person who wears it. In this chapter, I will address the factors that influence the "perfect" cut based on your individual features. These factors are body type, face shape, and facial features. These are obvious and important as you contemplate your overall look, yet they're all too often overlooked when women think about their hairstyle.

When you consider these factors as you design your new look with your stylist, you have the opportunity to enhance your best features and balance or harmonize your flaws. I don't talk about hiding flaws as the idea of flaws in the first place is, well, flawed. Our society values thinness, but not all societies do. If we don't have the "perfect" body according to others, rather than accepting who we are or trying to change it to fit our perception of a healthy body, we often will take drastic steps that endanger our health. We often want a quick fix to any area that could be altered with diet, exercise, or simple practices. There were times in the past when a voluptuous body was valued and considered beautiful. You can be sexy, attractive, and beautiful no matter your size; it is the way you feel about yourself and carry yourself (your attitude and carriage) that affect the way others perceive you. I always see something of striking beauty in each of my clients. It is my goal is to help my clients find the best way to achieve the look that expresses their confidence, energy, and beauty.

I notice my clients' body type whenever they walk toward me. It is critically important that your haircut be compatible with your body type. Look into a full-length mirror to get a clear view of your overall image, as this is what others see, not just your face. Turn to each side and study your body. Look at your back side as this is also on display and should be considered when cutting the back of your hair. Your face shape and facial features also play an important part in designing a haircut. I use my client's face shape to determine the length and shape of her haircut. The techniques I use are based on her elements. This chapter is about the integration of holistic influences or factors in determining you best haircut.

Determining Your Perfect Length

There is a perfect method that I use to determine the best hair length for your face and body type. In our salon, it is called the "one third" rule, which works as follows:

Tip: Your hair length should never be more than one third of your height.

Place your forefinger at the center point of your hairline at the top of your forehead. Extend your little finger to the corner of your eye in the temple area. This span between your forefinger and your little finger will be your base measurement and represents the first third.

Replicate this base measurement twice. The second third should take you to right above the jawline. The final third will take you to your ideal hair length.

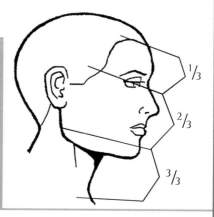

For a layered cut, the distance between the hairline and the perfect length is where the layers should start. To determine your ideal short hair length, take the midway point between the center point of your hairline and your ideal hair length.

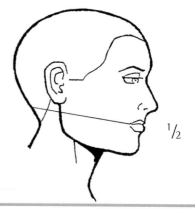

Body Type

Stand in front of a mirror and study your body type from the front, side, and back angle. You will get a truer picture if you observe yourself without any clothes on. It is important that you work with the body type you have right now, not the type you want to have, had in the past, or are working toward. This can be a difficult moment for many women, because they are trained to not be satisfied with their bodies. Try to step out of your critical analysis for a moment and be objective as you select which body type is most like what you see in the mirror. If it helps, pretend you are evaluating someone else's body. It is very easy to see if someone else has a "vertical" or "voluptuous" body type; it may be easier for you to see your own body type if you can be objective for a moment.

You'll notice that all of these body types are positive. Our body type is determined as much by genetics as by our habits, including diet and exercise, but our bodies are changing throughout our lives. If you've ever had children, you know what it's like to go through dramatic changes in a short time period, and you may experience permanent changes. But hairstyles change too! So work with what's right in front of you in the mirror, and come back as many times as you'd like for another look.

- Are you **vertical** with long limbs and a lean torso?
- Are you **curvaceous** with well-defined curves?
- Are you **muscular** with a V-shaped torso, broad shoulders, and little hip definition?
- Are you **curved**, which is similar to vertical but with more curves?
- Are you **voluptuous** with full features and wider curves?

The hair cuts that I recommend as being the best for each body type are:

Vertical: long limbs and lean torso
- Short hair: 90° with texture throughout
- Medium hair: Blunt or solid line, cut at midpoint between cheekbone and jawline
- Long hair: Horizontal lines from the crown to the end of the hair

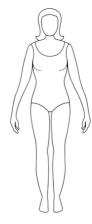

Curved: similar to vertical but with more curves

- Short: A 90° cut with texturized ends to show off movement
- Medium: Cut midway between the cheekbone and jawline for the best length or for the first cut in layering
- Long hair: Cut "U" shape in length plus lots of layering and texturizing for movement

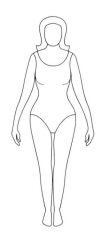

Curvaceous: well-defined curves

- Short hair: One and a half to two inches long, texturized to create movement and support
- Medium hair: A bob with layers to create soft volume and movement
- Long hair: Long layers to create movement

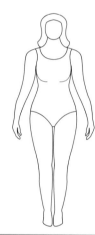

Muscular: V-shaped back, thicker torso, and little hip definition

- Short hair: Angled cuts with geometric lines with texture to add strength and height
- Medium hair: Layer to create free flowing ends
- Long hair: Cut "U" shape in length. Layer to create free flowing ends for softness

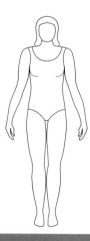

Voluptuous: full features with wider curves

- Short hair: Create height and angles, need movement plus soft volume and more angular lines
- Medium hair: Create layers and graduated height with little fullness
- Long hair: Same as curvaceous, long layers to create movement, hair should not cover more than one third of body

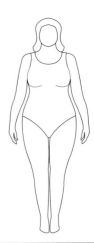

Face Shape

The second factor is face shape, which is sometimes hard to determine. Stand in front of the mirror with your hair combed straight back from your face. (This is easiest to do after washing your hair.) The oval face shape is considered the most ideal by many; however, it is important to honor your face shape. Many studies have shown that most people find symmetry attractive, and an oval face shape appears to be the most symmetrical of all face shapes. All of the tips that I have included about haircuts and coloring are designed to create the image of a symmetrical face shape. Placement of color is as important as choosing the right color and cut. The right placement creates an optical illusion of slimming, widening, elongating, or shortening the face. You need to recognize your own face shape in order to understand where to place colors in order to create a balanced face shape. Darkness slims and recedes while lightness increases size and accentuates. For more technical information on hair coloring according to your element, please see Chapter 12 and Appendix 1, which you can show to your stylist.

Oval

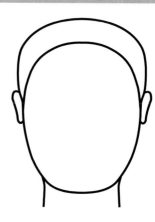

Face is round but slightly elongated. The jaw is as wide as the forehead.

Haircuts

Longer cuts are recommended, however, with an oval face shape, you may select any cut as long as you make certain to check with the suggestions for your body type and facial features.

Hair Color

Keep a half inch around hairline a solid color so not to change the face shape.

Heart

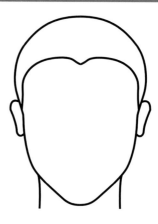

This is the most common face shape. The face has a wide forehead and draws to a point at the chin.

Haircuts

- Short cuts should be closer to the head from the temple to the jawline. Cut into the hair, creating artichoke textured effects and leaving more height in the crown area.
- Bobs should be layered.
- A medium length cut should be layered to create texture.
- Long cuts can be either layered or straight.
- For styling, side parts are best.
- Fringes (bangs) widen the face. If you desire fringes, make certain that they are long and sweep to the side. They should hit at the cheek level.

Hair Color

- Longer fringes that sweep to the side can be highlighted to add width as long as they drop below the cheek.
- For fringes across the forehead keep the outer corners darker, and place lighter pieces in the middle of the forehead.
- If you wear your hair parted in the middle, your highlights or lighter color must begin away from the forehead.
- Lighter colors will make the forehead appear wider so keep the color around the forehead darker.

Round

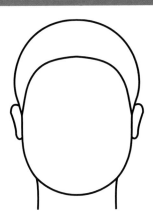

The face looks full and wide, as the distance between the lower lip and the end of the chin is short.

Haircuts
• You can wear a bob cut to the lip with no fringe.
• A short square cut will create height on top of head to lengthen the face.
• If you prefer medium to long hair, it needs to be layered to create balance.

Hair Color
• Kepp the area from the top of your ears forward darker.
• Keep fringes darker, if you have them.
• Keep a half inch around hairline darker to slenderize the face.
• Add highlights to the center of the head to add height.

Square

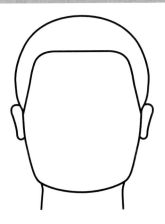

The face has a strong, angular jawline and wide forehead.

Haircuts
• A short cut should be layered with fringes sweeping to one side.
• The cut should have a horizontal, round shape to counter the vertical, square shape in order to lengthen the face.
• Medium to long cuts with a graduated fringe in front create movement to offset the square shape.
• A vertical cut line will offset a horizontal jawline and make the face appear slimmer.
• You can wear fringes that sweep to one side or center parts.

Hair Color
• Keep the outside corners of fringes darker or a solid color.
• For a middle part (which slims the width of a square forehead), add highlights or lighten your color at the center point of your forehead.
• For fringes that sweep at the temple, highlight or lighten the cheek area.

Oblong

The oblong face is equal in width from forehead to jawline, with a more linear appearance than an oval face.

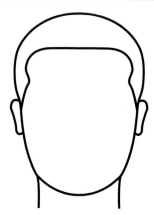

Haircuts
- Short cuts are recommended.
- Keep fringes longer to cover forehead.
- Layered bobs styled with flips or lots of texture for fullness are recommended.

Hair Color
- Color fringes darker to shorten the face.
- Add lighter colors in the area from the ear to the temple area to add width.
- If your hair is styled with flips or kicked-out pieces, add highlights to that area to add width.
- For side sweep fringes, add width with highlights.

Diamond

The face has a narrow chin, wider through the cheek area.

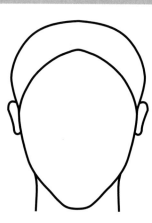

Haircuts
- Short cuts with fringes are preferable.
- Medium lengths should be layered and styled away from the face to open the face at the temples.
- Long lengths should be sleek with fringes or have long layers.

Hair Color
- With color, the goal is to create lightness or highlights to add width to the narrow forehead.
- Add depth to the sides in front of the ear to slenderize the cheek area.
- Behind the ear, add highlights to add width to a narrow jaw.

Facial Features (Facial Triangle)

Now that you are aware of your face shape and the haircuts that I recommend for each shape, the next step is consideration for facial features. I call this the facial triangle and divide the face into thirds when considering hair cuts. The idea is to enhance great features and to balance the cut in order to diminish any problem area.

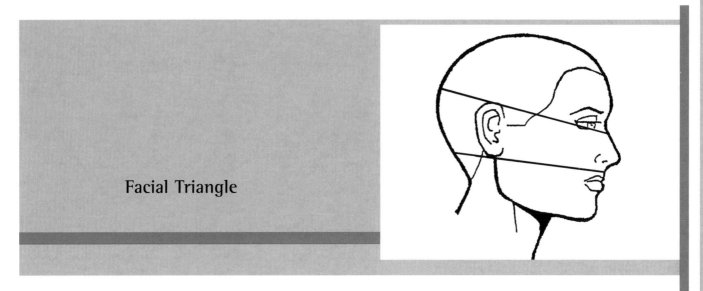

Facial Triangle

Top Third

Forehead
The forehead defines your hair line and serves as a determining factor regarding everything from fringe (bang) decisions to the length of your hair.
- Narrow: Cuts should be off and away from the forehead to open this area.
- Deep: Some fringes or bangs will minimize the forehead and can be swept to one side according to face shape.

Eyebrows
Eyebrows can be adjusted easily with shaping or color. Make certain your eyebrows coordinate with your hair color. They are usually a shade or two darker than your hair color.
- Shape: Arch and density must be considered when selecting upper contour of the hair cut.
- Glasses should never be wider than widest part of face and should never go above the eyebrow.

Eyes

The eyes have been called the mirror of the soul. They are one of your most expressive features. Eyes are always unique and beautiful, and it's from your eye color and skin tone that your true colors will be determined.

- Large eyes: Short hair will frame and accentuate large eyes. If you wear your hair longer, pull it away from your face to show your eyes.
- Small eyes: Be careful so hair does not overpower smaller eyes.

Middle Third

Nose

The nose is a very prominent feature of the face as it is the center. In America, people are more self-conscious about our noses than people are in other countries.

- Prominent: Fringes need to be left full in order to balance. Create fullness in the fringe area around the hair line.
- Small: Short cuts look great if face shape allows; hair should not appear too full as your face will not appear balanced.

Cheekbones

Your cheekbones add shape and angles to your face. If you have nice, high cheekbones, you don't want to cover them, you want to showcase them.

- Soft: Your hair should be cut or styled to brush back from your face. You can also accentuate your cheekbones with makeup to make them appear stronger.
- Hard: Short cuts work well by enhancing strong cheekbones; softening this feature will dramatically alter your overall appearance.

Ears

The ears are the halfway point on your face.

- Large: Cuts should be longer to cover at least the upper half of the ear. If hair is too short for coverage, make sure the hair is textured to shift focus away from the ears.
- Small: It is important to balance your face shape with your haircut. With small ears, you can wear most haircuts. You may want to accentuate the ears by styling your hair so they will show.

Bottom Third

Lips

People watch your lips as you speak. They draw the eyes and attention to your face. Lips are very easily enhanced or balanced with the proper lipstick colors, application, and lip liner.

- Full: Any cut works well with the ideal lip shape. If your face shape permits, you may want the cut or layer to begin at your lip line. This will draw attention to your lips.
- Small: Small lips can be changed with makeup techniques.

Chin and Jaw

The jawline is the frame of the face. It is one of the defining features for you face shape.

- Soft: Cuts that have lines at the jawline will help accentuate a soft line.
- Strong: Geometric cuts accentuate the jawline. The cut line should fall above or below the jawline.

Neck

The length and width of the neck are very important in determining hair length.

- Long: Medium length cuts should be used to balance a long neck; shorter cuts should flick outward and be colored lighter. If you want to emphasize a longer neck, style your hair so it is way from your face or pulled back.
- Short: Hair should be slightly above midway to give the illusion of length.
- Thick: A cut with soft lines will balance your look. Avoid a square cut; the cut should emphasize softness, not a blunt line.

These are the holistic factors, or the outside characteristics, that play a vital role in determining the correct hairstyle for your face shape, body type, and facial features. Feng Shui is used to determine the techniques that make these hair cuts unique for you. If you are a Fire/Earth Yin Moderate 4 with a vertical body type, square face shape, small eyes, small nose, and long neck, your haircut will be different than someone with a Fire/Earth Yin Moderate 4 with a voluptuous body type, round face shape, large eyes, prominent nose, and thick neck. My desire is to assist you in creating a haircut and hairstyle designed by you, for you.

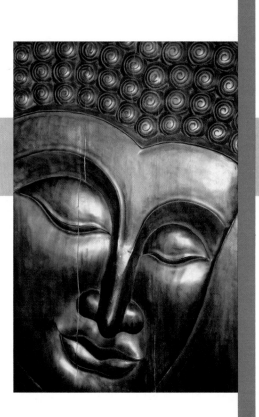

12 Skin Tone and Hair Color

Color has been an influence on our lives since we were born. From birth, we have responded to different colors. Some colors speak to us, some excite us, and some calm us. Color is also a way to identify ourselves; to show our personality in our home, wardrobe, and hair. Specific colors are often identified with special occasions such as red for Valentine's Day, white for weddings, red and green for Christmas, or blue for the birth of a boy and pink for a girl. In Feng Shui, the five elements have certain characteristics that are associated with them, including colors. Yin energy represents cool colors and Yang energy represents warm colors.

How does color influence our life-world? First, color defines for us what exists and what does not exist. Second, color discloses the status of one's health and fortunes, thus traditional Chinese doctors are versed in reading the color of one's face or one's Chi. Third, color inspires emotion. We feel upbeat and satisfied if the status of our Chi matches the color of our clothes. When in low spirits, for example, we shun red apparel. Fourth, color also structures our behavior. The force that links us with color is Chi.

Respecting the fact that each person is an individual and temple, the elements will help define who you are and how far you are willing to express yourself through color. A person who is truly in balance has a presence of all five elements in her life. Most people have one or two dominant elements, but they should be aware of the remaining elements in order to help incorporate them into their lifestyle. This assists in creating true balance; emotionally, physically, and holistically.

Skin Tone

The theory of absorption and reflection describes how colors react to each other. Two colors placed next to each other have a reaction; either absorption or reflection. For example; if your eye color is blue-gray and blue eye shadow is placed on your lids, the blues of the eyes and the shadow absorb into one another and reflect more of the gray in the eye color. If gray eye shadow is used, the eyes will reflect more blue. Based on this theory, the choice of hair color and color of clothing that is directly next to the face is very important. You should wear colors that compliment your skin tone and eye color. Understanding your skin tone and then incorporating it with the color wheel along with the absorption and reflection theory will enable you to choose the hair color, makeup, and clothing that will work best for you.

To find your correct skin tone look at your face—not your arms nor the inside of your wrist. The exposure to the sun causes the arms to have much more color than the face. Also understand that with exposure to the sun, the skin tone will change to a warmer palette. This is a template only, of course; there are exceptions to these broad categories. If you do not fit into these categories, you should follow your actual skin tone. You will notice in the following descriptions of skin tones that I sometimes make reference to cool or warm. Use the skin tone color wheel as a reference point.

To keep the skin tones as simple as possible, the first division is light or dark eyes. Light eyes include families that are blue, gray, turquoise, green, blue green, green yellow, hazel with green, or hazel with yellow. Dark eyes are brown, brown with gold, brown with red, hazel with brown, hazel with green, black, or hazel with golden. There are two light skin tone families; porcelain and milky. There are three dark skin tones; honey, olive, and ebony. The skin tones as well as eye color are divided into warm and cool skin tones. I am listing the eye colors that are generally associated with the skin tones.

Light Skin Tones

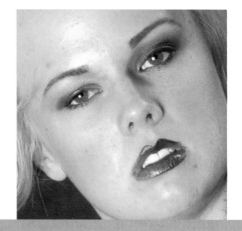

Porcelain Skin Tone

This is a cool skin tone that has the presence of pink undertones in the skin and generally has light, cool eye coloring such as blue, gray, blue gray, or turquoise.

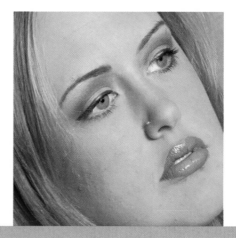

Milky Skin Tone

This is a warm skin tone that has the presence of an ivory, creamy undertone with the eyes being warmer on the light side: green, hazel with green, or blue-green.

Dark Skin Tones

Honey Skin Tone

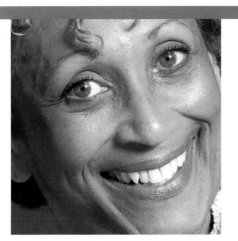

Honey has the presence of golden-bronze undertones of warmth in the skin with the eye coloring of brown, brown-red, brown with golden, or black.

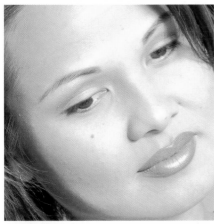

Olive Skin Tone

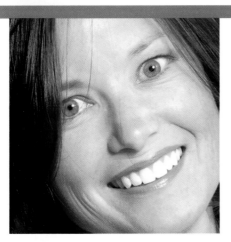

Olive has the presence of a green cool undertone and the absence of warmth, with eye coloring of hazel with green, or brown with red. With sun exposure, this skin tone tans very easily and then becomes Honey.

Ebony Skin Tone

Ebony is the skin tone of African Americans and has cool dark undertones. Eye color is usually black. African American skin with more light golden tones is classified as Honey.

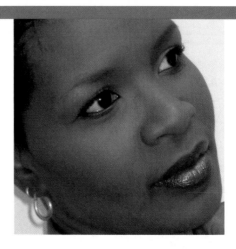

Ruby Skin Tone

Ruby is any skin tone with the excess presence of red. The red comes from the capillaries near the surface of the skin.

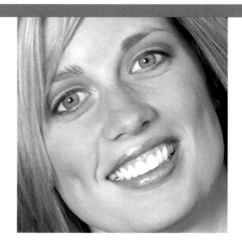

Your True Colors

The skin tone color wheel shows your "true" color. Your skin tone and eye color should guide you as to which colors are your true best colors to wear in hair color, makeup, and clothing.

It's interesting that people may be attracted to colors that are not their best colors. Finding out what your best colors are does not mean you have to replace your wardrobe completely. Use the colors you're attracted to as accent colors in accessories, patterns, or one piece of your outfit, while having the outfit predominantly in the colors that suit you best. These are your true colors; stay true to them.

Skin Tone Color Wheel

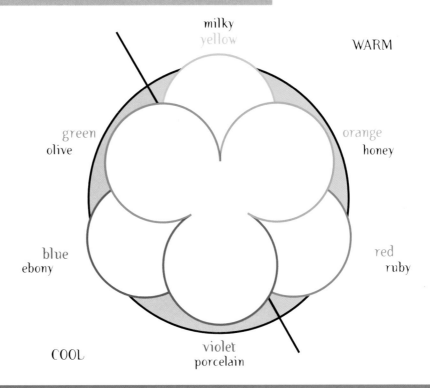

milky
yellow

WARM

green
olive

orange
honey

blue
ebony

red
ruby

COOL

violet
porcelain

Porcelain skin is the cool tone with pink undertones and cool eye color. This skin type looks best in white, black, purple, light blue, or a pastel color palette for wardrobe. In hair color, cool blondes are known as ash or platinum. Cool brown colors such as light ash brown look best. Red hair color has to be a very true red-red color, not red on the warm side—no orange tone. Silver or platinum jewelry reflect best on porcelain skin.

Milky skin is the warm tone with ivory or creamy undertones with warm eye color. Milky skin looks the best in cream, off-white, ivory, orange, brown, tan, or tangerine colors of clothing. Gold jewelry looks the best. In hair color, warm blondes are known as golden blonde or copper blonde. Warm browns are known as auburn or golden brown.

Honey skin is the warm tone with a golden bronze undertone. The wardrobe colors that look the best are browns, khaki, camel, and cream. Hair color for blondes will have golden or copper tones. Browns are warm browns such as golden with auburn or orange. Jewelry should be gold with lots of warmth.

Olive skin tone is the cool tone with a cool green undertone. Olive skin tones look best in rich cool jewel tones in their wardrobe. Rich berry, sapphire blue, and evergreen colors look great on olive skin. Cool blondes are known as ash blonde or platinum blonde. Brown hair on the cool side has ash or green-blue tones. Reds are the burgundy, rich berry reds. Silver and platinum jewelry look the best.

Ebony skin is cool and reflects colors that are very true. Strong, bold shades of every color are fabulous; orange-orange, red-red, violet, and true strong pinks are great. Hair color needs to be kept rich and dark on the cool side: dark violets or dark cool reds. Platinum or silver jewelry, or jewelry with bold colors look best.

Ruby skin tone has excessive redness which is caused from capillaries close to the surface. The object with the wardrobe and hair color is to cool the skin. Ash browns or ash blondes look best on hair. Khaki green, tan, or black looks best on skin. The object is no red or red-oranges. Keep the warmth away from the skin.

True Color vs. Complementary Color

The previous information is based on the true colors for each skin tone. The true color comes from identifying the skin tone and hair color tones from the color wheels shown. The color wheel is divided into warm and cool. Ying is cool and Yang is warm. All hair color, makeup, and clothing companies have color palettes based on this color wheel. With the addition of white, the color is lightened; the addition of dark such as gray or black deepens the color. When you mix the three primaries together you will produce a neutral brown tone.

When you use a cool color versus a warm color, go directly across the color wheel—that is your complementary color. Cool blue is directly across from warm orange. Warm yellow is directly across from cool violet. If your skin is milky, your hair color is a golden blonde, and you are wearing a lavender or purple blouse, your true color is warm (skin and hair) and you are wearing complementary cool violet. The "absorb and reflect" theory is that your skin and hair are going to appear a buttery flawless color and the clothing is going to stand out. When the skin and hair are both a true palette, you can accessorize with complementary colors and it looks great. If your skin is one tone and your hair is a complementary color such as honey skin tone and a violet hair color, you need to change the tones of your makeup foundation so that your skin does not reflect an excess yellow. The hair color and skin tone are reflecting each other as opposites do and they reflect excessively.

Color Formula Wheel

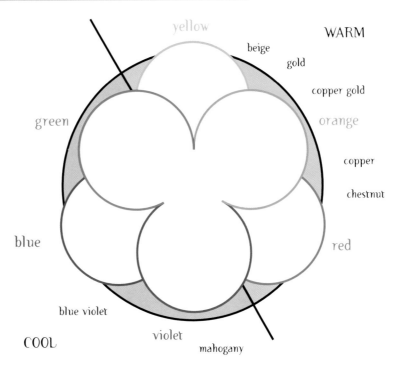

Hair Color

When referring to a hair color, it is known as "tone." There are many romantic color names in the color world. Instead of green tones in the hair, it is fluffed to "ash" or represented by a letter A. Numbers are also assigned such as 3=Green because most consumers are afraid of Green hair when green is actually essential in hair coloring. It controls excess red tones found in naturally dark hair colors. The good news is that you are not limited to one hair color. The thing to remember is that the tone of the color must work with your skin tone. As long as you have true skin and hair colors, you can accessorize with complementary colors.

Our hair color formulations are based on your skin tone, natural hair level, and element. The first number of the color listed in the Schwarzkopf color chart represents hair level. Determine what your natural hair level is by comparing your hair to the sample pictured on pages 186 and 187. The second number on the chart represents the tone of the color. Refer to the Color Formula Wheel to see the colors designated as warm or cool tones. True colors for warm skin tones such as Milky and Honey are Beige, Gold, Auburn, Copper, Copper Gold, and Chestnut. True colors for cool skin tones such as Porcelain, Olive, and Ebony are Ash, Smokey, Matt, Natural, Violet Ash, and Mahogany. Schwarzkopf uses numbers whereas other color lines will use names for their color tones. These color strands are from the manufacturer whose color we use in our salons.

Element:

Fire
Your skin tone is the only determining factor for your choice of hair colors. You can be as daring as you wish.

Earth
Find your natural hair level. If you are a level 5, you may select colors from two levels down [level 3 or 4] or two levels up [level 6 or 7]. Your skin tone will determine whether you select warm color tones or cool color tones.

Metal
Find your natural hair level. If you are a level 6, you may select colors from three levels down [level 3, 4, or 5] or four levels up [level 7, 8, 9, or 10]. Your skin tone will determine whether you select warm color tones or cool color tones.

Water
Find your natural hair level. If you are a natural level 5, you may select colors from four levels down [level 1, 2, 3, or 4] or five levels up [level 6, 7, 8, 9, or 10]. Your skin tone will determine whether you select cool or warm color tones.

Wood
Find your natural hair level. If you are a natural level 6, you may select colors from two levels down [level 4 or 5] or three levels up [level 7, 8, or 9]. You skin tone will determine whether you select cool or warm color tones.

Follow your Skin Tone guide for your best tonal color. Follow your Element guide for your best color selection.

IGORA ROYAL

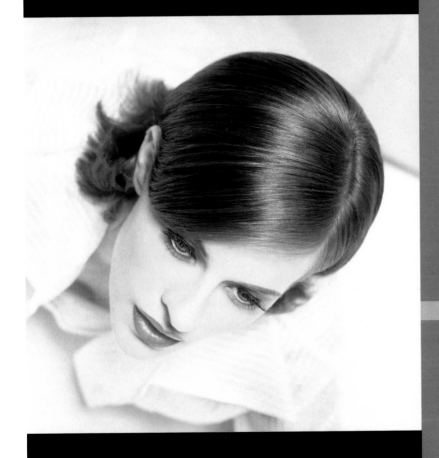

COLOR GUIDE

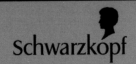

Schwarzkopf

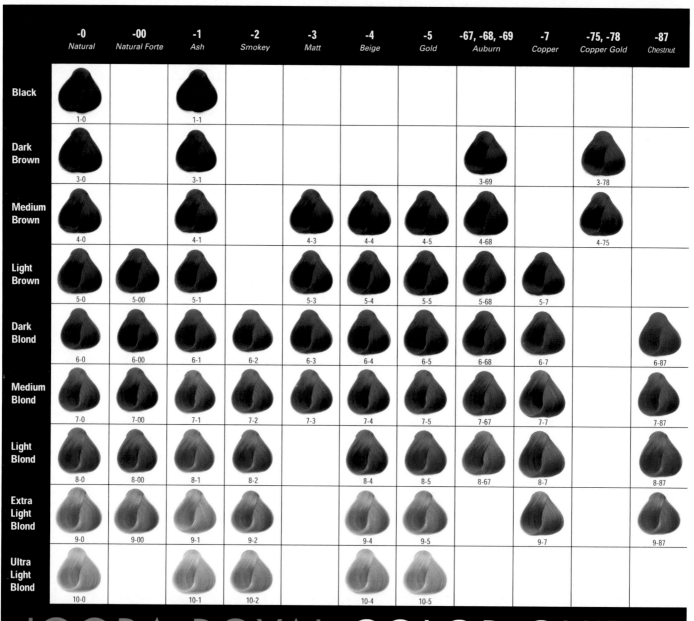

	-0 Natural	-00 Natural Forte	-1 Ash	-2 Smokey	-3 Matt	-4 Beige	-5 Gold	-67, -68, -69 Auburn	-7 Copper	-75, -78 Copper Gold	-87 Chestnut
Black	1-0		1-1								
Dark Brown	3-0		3-1					3-69		3-78	
Medium Brown	4-0		4-1		4-3	4-4	4-5	4-68		4-75	
Light Brown	5-0	5-00	5-1		5-3	5-4	5-5	5-68	5-7		
Dark Blond	6-0	6-00	6-1	6-2	6-3	6-4	6-5	6-68	6-7		6-87
Medium Blond	7-0	7-00	7-1	7-2	7-3	7-4	7-5	7-67	7-7		7-87
Light Blond	8-0	8-00	8-1	8-2		8-4	8-5	8-67	8-7		8-87
Extra Light Blond	9-0	9-00	9-1	9-2		9-4	9-5		9-7		9-87
Ultra Light Blond	10-0		10-1	10-2		10-4	10-5				

IGORA ROYAL COLOR GUIDE

-88 Mahogany	-10 Blonding Shades	-91 Violet Ash	Ultimate High Lifts	Concentrates	
					Black
		9.5-5	12-0	0-10	**Dark Brown**
		9.5-7	11-1	0-11	**Medium Brown**
5-88		9.5-91	11-2	0-22	**Light Brown**
6-88	6-10		11-4	0-33	**Dark Blond**
7-88	7-10			0-55	**Medium Blond**
	8-10			0-77	**Light Blond**
				0-88	**Extra Light Blond**
				0-99	**Ultra Light Blond**

Schwarzkopf

Coloring Techniques for the Elements

Share this information with your stylist to bring out your element with hair color.

Fire Techniques

- Your only limitations for hair color are your skin tone and personal preference.
- Place opposite colors right next to one another such as Platinum Blonde with Golden or Copper, Red and Berry Red.
- Create definite patterns such as squares and triangles that are lighter or darker.
- Put large pieces of different colors such as level one black with a level ten blonde on long choppy pieces; very Picasso.
- Hoshi-Star: make star pattern at crown cowlick; lighten or darken the remaining hair.
- Panel: make panel square patterns, five going around the Vertical Panel (VP), alternate colors. On the Horizontal Panel (HP) apply different color in five sections.

Earth Techniques

- You may select colors from two levels down from your natural level to two levels up. For example, if you are level six, you may select from levels four through eight.
- La Luna: Circular shapes. On the top crown zigzag out a circular pattern—top area lighter, the bottom area darker. The face shape will determine whether or not you keep the perimeter one inch around the face light or dark, (if round, darken; if diamond, lighten; etc. See Chapter 11 for more details on highlight placement for facial shape.)
- Chose a semi-permanent color (one that will fade out), follow panel application, and adjust for face shape with a zigzag part for a natural progression.

Metal Techniques

- You may select colors from three levels down from your natural level to four levels up. If you are a level six, this would mean you could choose from levels three trough ten.
- Use very small zigzag patterns in a halo pattern around face and gradually fade to no color in division C.
- Use two, three, or four colors with levels such as nine, eight and seven. (Two to three rows of level nine, two to three rows of level eight and two to three rows of level seven.)

Water Techniques

- You may select colors from four levels down from your natural level to five levels up. If you are a level six, this would mean you may select from levels two through eleven.
- Monet techniques: Start in nape, take zigzag one inch subsection alternating three different colors in the same family. Randomly place colors in each subsection and work your way up the head.

- Water weave patterns should show color separation between colors: a light color seen with a dark to medium next to it. As the foils process you can add another color to the remaining hair outside of foils.
- Diamond shape weave pattern: section top head area into diamond shape, adjust the diamond point according to face shape (forward for oval or square, backward for round or heart shape). Slice using lightest color around diamond outside shape, work inward with next lighter color then lighter than second color. Follow up with all-over color to remaining hair.

Wood Techniques

- You may select colors from two levels down from your natural level or three levels up. If you are a natural six, you may select from levels four through nine.
- Soft progression of colors—light, medium, to dark—zigzag part divisions A-B-C, with A lightest, B medium, C dark.
- To show a definite difference use two levels difference, if you want a softer blend use one level difference.
- Do a Wood weave piece pickup, then shampoo out weave, and apply a color to entire head to create a natural highlight tone effect.

Element	Fire	Earth	Metal	Water	Wood
Color	Artistic	Natural	Elegant classic	Elegant chic	Sporty
Techniques	Slice, Tokyo highlights	4-6 pieces weave	7-9 pieces weave	2-7 pieces weave	4-4 pieces weave
	2-4 colors used	2-4 colors used	1-2-3 colors used	1-2-3 colors used	2-3 colors used
	Anything goes in level range	2 up 2 down level range	4 up 3 down level range	5 up 4 down level range	3 up 2 down level range

For more information or support with these techniques, please call Yamaguchi Enterprises at (800) 572-5661.

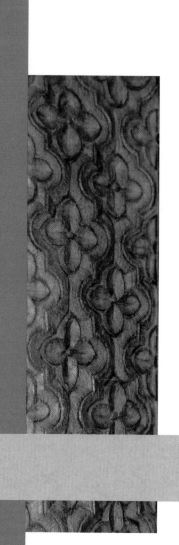

13 Makeup

Makeup is a fun accessory—something you can change as your mood or element strikes you. Change from day to evening, spring to fall, Earth to Water, or Water to Fire. But keep in mind, makeup should be used as an enhancement, not as a cover. I want to see my clients' faces! I want to see their cheekbones, their true nose shapes, their skin color. I understand the desire to cover up skin flaws, but you don't need to cover up your face with excess makeup. I want and need to see my guests' true skin, and your friends and loved ones want to see your true face, too!

In this chapter on makeup, I will share with you the proper makeup colors according to skin tone and element. I'll also share tips with you on the proper brushes and how to use them, sharing techniques according to each element.

But all the makeup techniques and ideas I share with you will be worthless if you don't take proper care of your skin. What you consume has a major impact on how healthy your skin looks, so healthy eating is a must, along with exercise, meditation, and rest. Vitamins and minerals help your skin as well. At least two to three pints of clean, pure water must be drunk daily, and alcoholic beverages consumed in moderation, as alcohol causes dehydration, depriving the skin of precious moisture. Smoking is damaging to the skin, as are UV rays. These are the two major causes of premature skin aging. Wear sunscreen with at least SPF 15 daily and reapply as needed. Choose your skin care products with care. Read the ingredients and demand the cleanest for your skin. Of course, cleanse your face every morning and night.

Using your healthy skin as a canvas, makeup will look wonderful. Since makeup is not a permanent application, you can go ahead and experiment. Have fun with it!

Colors have an absorption and reflection theory, the same as hair color. Colors absorb one another and reflect each other so you need to be aware of this concept. One example is if you have blue gray eye coloring and you wear blue eye shadow, the two blues absorb each other and the eye will reflect a more gray tone. If you wear gray eye shadow, the grays absorb and eyes will reflect a more blue tone.

Makeup should be fun and experimental. Most women have worn their makeup the same way for years. Although the colors may change, the application does not. Makeup is something that should change whether it is color, application, or technique, because our features and skin change as we age.

In order to analyze your skin, look in the mirror and evaluate your facial skin, not arm skin. Don't rely on what you have been told in the past. If you are of Hispanic, Japanese, or Italian ethnicity, you need to select the correct skin tone and not just assume that you are olive because you have been told in the past that that is your skin tone. You could be olive, honey, or ruby depending on the color that is in the reflection.

Porcelain

Porcelain skin tone is very light with pink undertones. The skin does not tan, but it usually burns very easily when exposed to the sun. The eye color is usually blue, gray, turquoise, blue with yellow or blue with gray.

Your true colors for makeup are pinks, purples, mauve, grays, and blues. Your true wardrobe colors or best colors are white, black, pinks, purples, and blues. Your complementary or balancing colors are colors that you can use in your accessories such as scarves, pins, or belts. These colors are: yellows, greens, peaches, creams, browns, and oranges. When you choose to wear complementary colors in your wardrobe, you should adjust your makeup colors to complementary.

Milky

Milky skin tone has a creamy, peachy undertone with eye coloring that is green, hazel with green, hazel with golden brown, green with yellow, or green with brown. This skin tone does tan after slow, continuous exposure to the sun.

Your true colors for makeup are greens, golds, peaches, and browns. Your true wardrobe colors are creams, beiges, tans, camels, browns, greens, yellows, and turquoise. The complementary makeup colors are pinks, mauves, blues, and purples. Complementary wardrobe colors are pinks, blues, black, and white.

Honey

Honey skin tone is the presence of bronze and gold warmth. This skin tone tans very easily. The eye color is brown, hazel with green, hazel with brown, brown black, red brown, and brown with golden.

The true colors in makeup are browns, golds, rusts, and oranges. True wardrobe colors are creams, browns, red-oranges, cinnamon, golds, red-browns, and oranges. (Think warm colors.)

Complementary makeup colors are grays, navy, blues, berries, black, or forest green. Complementary wardrobe colors are black, white, burgundy, red-reds, and blues. (Think cool colors.)

Olive

Olive skin tone has a green, cool undertone and the absence of yellow or warmth. Eye color will be brown, hazel with green, brown, gold, red-brown, brown-brown, or brown-black.

True makeup colors are black, gray, berries, red-red, and violets. True wardrobe colors are pinks, blues, black, gray, white, berries, and khaki.

Complementary makeup colors are gold, brown, and rust. Complementary wardrobe colors are cream, browns, gold, and cinnamon.

Ebony

Ebony skin tone is black—no presence of golden, but dark. This skin has a cool reflection with the true color. It is best with bright true pigments such as pinks, blues, berries, fuchsia, and other jewel tones.

Complementary colors in makeup are gold, bronzes, and rust. Complementary wardrobe colors are oranges and yellows.

Because of the darkness of this skin tone, bright vibrant pigments, whether true or complementary, look best.

Ruby

Ruby is the presence of red in the skin due capillaries close to the skin surface. Because any of the other skin tones can change to Ruby, this tone corresponds with all eye colors. The object is to cool the skin with the use of green concealers under the foundation.

The Color Wheel

When you understand your skin tone, the color wheel helps explain the true colors. The complementary colors are located directly across the wheel.

True colors are colors that blend and work well with your skin tone. The colors work together to absorb and reflect the skin tone: rosy pink with Porcelain, peachy ivory with Milky, golden with Honey, creamy with Olive, and all colors reflect very dark with Ebony. When you choose an opposite makeup color application, expect the skin tone to appear more intense and eye color to pop.

Skin Tone Color Wheel

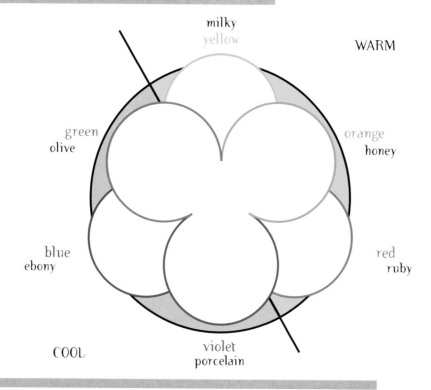

milky
yellow

WARM

green
olive

orange
honey

blue
ebony

red
ruby

COOL

violet
porcelain

Makeup Color Tips

- If you have Porcelain skin with blue gray eyes, use a bit of gold and orange as eyeliners.
- If you have Milky skin tone with green eyes, use a bit of violet, blue-violet, red-violet, or fuchsia eyeliners.
- If you have Honey skin tone with brown eyes, use blue to blue-violet or blue-green eyeliners.
- If you have Olive skin tone with brown or hazel eyes, use rust, orange, or red-orange eyeliners.
- If you have Ebony skin tone with black eyes, use orange, gold, or red-orange eyeliners.

When incorporating complementary colors in your wardrobe and makeup, the clothing and makeup absorb into each other and the skin tone will reflect with more color true to its undertones. Porcelain will appear pinker to purple, Milky more yellow, Honey more golden yellow, Olive greener, Ebony more black-blue.

A daytime application should be a more natural, lighter application while an evening application is more dramatic, with more color on the eyes and lips. During the day, if the eye shadow application is dramatic and strong, the lips are more neutral and played down. With evening application, you can use drama in both features.

Some people like the complementary reflection. I recommend the hair be a true color to the skin; use makeup and clothing (temporary accessories) as fun complementary colors for a change of pace. If you choose complementary color for your hair color, your makeup must be adjusted with concealers so your skin does not reflect too much color such as too much pink or gold.

Seasons

Makeup should be adjusted two times a year. Spring brings lighter, brighter colors to clothing, and makeup should be the same. Lighter, brighter shadows and lip tones should be more of a daytime natural application in the spring and summer time. Makeup should become a little deeper, with richer tones, in the fall and winter just as the clothing colors get deeper and darker. The hues are deeper so shadows and lips can become deeper, richer, more jewel-toned.

If your skin color changes in the summer from exposure to the sun, you will want to change your makeup color palette. For example, Olive skin tones may become very golden and warm as opposed to its natural cool tones, so it becomes necessary to change the cool palette to the warm colors for Honey skin tones because of the change in skin pigment—the addition of warmth.

Porcelain skin will tan with a slow and continuous application of exposure so you may be Porcelain as a true color but become Milky as the skin pigment warms. The makeup colors would change from Porcelain cool to Milky warm. The Porcelain colors will become your complementary colors.

Fire

Go more expressive with your colors.

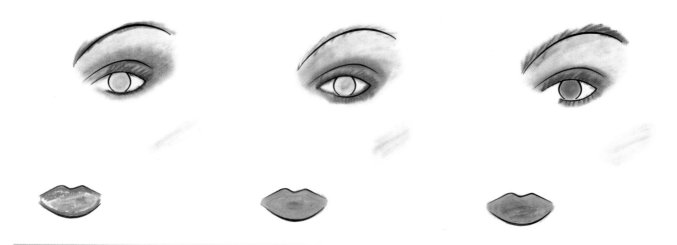

Porcelain

Emphasize the eyes with a gray or blue eyeliner and blue or purple shadows. Use deeper shades of purple or sparkling pinks on lips.

Milky

Think shiny with golds, rich auburn, and shades of browns and sparkly greens on eyes. Lips should be moist with nudes and peaches.

Honey

Use strong oranges, cinnamon, brown fall colors, or complementary strong pinks on eyes and lips. Use a shimmer across cheekbones.

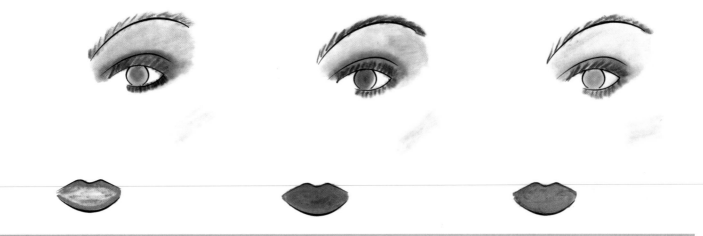

Olive
Create strong smoky eyes with soft colors such as mauve, gray, or black. For lips, use berry colors.

Ebony
Go for bold, strong jewel eye colors. Use berry, deep red, or orange on the lips.

Ruby
For sultry eyes, use a brown, gold, and rust along with gold, rust, and browns on the lips.

Makeup Techniques for Your Element

Earth

You'll want shades that look and feel natural to you.

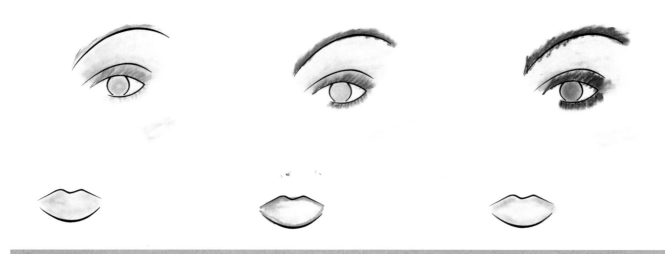

Porcelain
Use a light dusting of mauve to pink on eyelid and soft pink, sheer lip gloss.

Milky
Wear soft peach and ivory on eyelids with nude on your lips.

Honey
Wear soft browns on lids and soft nude to brown on your lips.

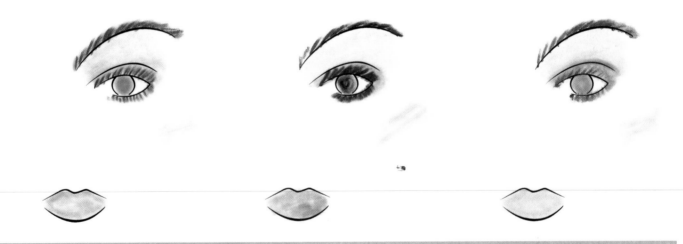

Olive
Use soft mauve, sheer shadow with an airbrush application, and keep lips mauve *au natural* shades.

Ebony
Wear a brown shadow and a brown, brick, or nude lip color.

Ruby
Use natural ivory or brown eye shadow and wear nude lips.

Makeup Techniques for Your Element

Metal

You'll want a look that's classic and subtle.

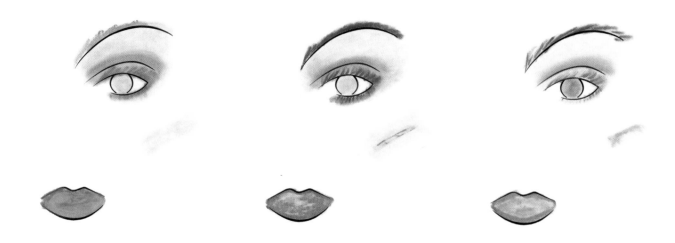

Porcelain
Eye shadow should be bone white, pink, mauve, lavender, or blue gray with brown to gray eyeliner. Wear lips mauve to pink.

Milky
Use browns to line lids and wear with ivory to peach shadows. Lips should be more peach to nude brown.

Honey
Wear brown liner with brown eye shadow. You can add ivory or cream to lids. Try rust lips to brown to nude depending on the season.

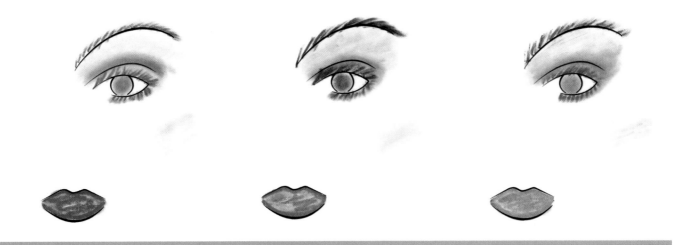

Olive
Wear russet red-brown or mauve shadow and berry lip color.

Ebony
Use russet red-brown shadow and brown red on lips.

Ruby
Use a brown liner for smoky eyes. Lips should be a brown or berry color.

Water
Go for a chic, fashion-forward look.

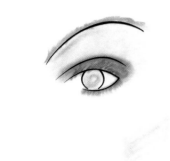

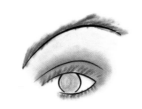

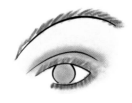

Porcelain
Wear bone white or blue gray eye shadows, lined with gray blue. Keep lips nude to pink.

Milky
Charcoal line the eyes and wear peach or warm brown eye shadow. Lips should be peach to nude to rust.

Honey
Achieve smoky brown eyes with rusts and gold eye shadow, and wear lips red-orange.

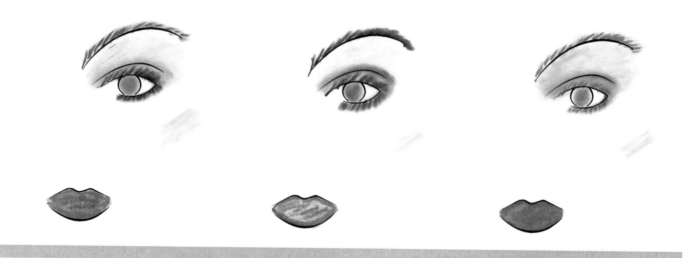

Olive
Use black or gray liners with berry or burgundy shadows. Berry or deep red should be on lips.

Ebony
Use strong smoky colors on eyes and berry or russet browns on lips.

Ruby
Wear flat browns, ivory, cream, and a hint of green on eyes, while keeping lips more brown to red.

Wood

You're going to want a natural look that doesn't interfere with all your activities.

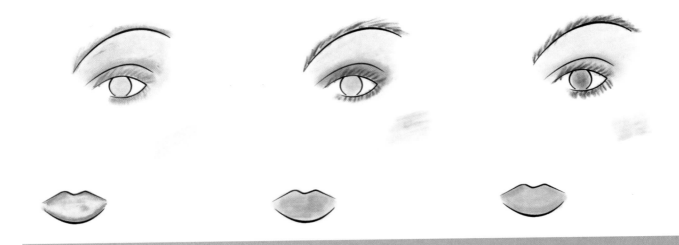

Porcelain
Wear a soft shimmer of pink dusted across lids and pink to nude lip gloss.

Milky
Use ivory and brown shadow with nude to peach lip gloss.

Honey
Wear shades of brown shadow with peach to brownish lips.

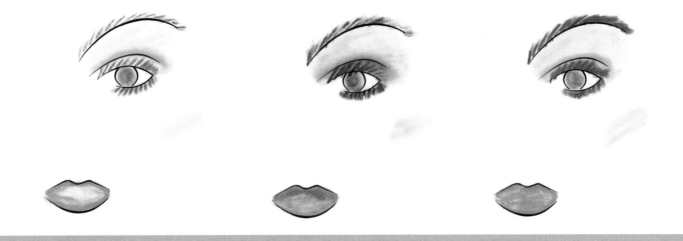

Olive
Use a light brush of berry on lids and mauve to pink lip gloss.

Ebony
Orange, reds, and browns should be worn on eyes and the lips.

Ruby
Wear bone or nude brown on the eyes and nude on the lips.

Makeup Application

In makeup application, there are different techniques. The use of a small makeup brush for the shadow creates more of specific placement of color. A larger brush creates an airbrush or softer application of color placement.

A face powder brush, being the largest, doesn't leave a line of demarcation. An eyeliner brush, being one of the smallest, gives more definition of the line. If you want a softer, more smudged line on eyes, use a larger brush. A blush brush is larger than a shadow brush, but smaller than face powder brushes so you get color placement but not too much concentration of color.

Makeup Techniques

Contouring

Heart
• Apply shading around the corners of the forehead and to the base of the chin.

Oval
• Apply shading on the corners of the forehead and corners of the jawline.

Round
• Contour vertically on sides of face to elongate the face.

Square
• Apply shading on the corners of the forehead and corners of the jawline.

Oblong
• Apply shading along the temples, the entire chin, and the jawline.

Diamond
• Apply shading to the top of the forehead, sides of the cheeks or temples, and the bottom of the chin.

Eyes
• To enlarge small eyes, use a lighter shade or shimmer only on the lower lid. Eyeliners should be used minimally.
• Accentuate the inner corners of wide-set eyes with darker colors, blending outward.

- For Asian eyes, if the upper lid is large, add depth to brow protrusion and highlight the brow bone. If the upper lid is small, apply dark shadow on the lower lid and smudge.
- On close-set eyes, use a lighter shade or no color on the inner half and blend a darker shade to the outside half.
- Use a highlighter all over the lids of deep-set eyes. Blend medium shade on the brow bone protrusion to add depth.
- Accentuate droopy eyes by applying shadow almost like cat's eyes. Take a final sweep upward on the outer corners.

Cheeks

Heart
- Apply blush from the apples of the cheek bones to the bottom of the ears.

Oval
- Apply blush right below the cheek bone to the top of the ear.

Round
- Apply blush in a forty-five degree angle from the apple of the cheek to the top of the ear.

Square
- Apply blush just below the cheek bone in a sixty degree angle up to the top of the ear.

Oblong and Diamond
- Apply blush on the cheek bone to the middle of the ear.

Lips
- For small lips, use a lighter shade or shimmer. Lip liner should be one to two shades darker than the lipstick.
- Use a matte shade and/or a luster shade for full lips.
- Use a lip liner to draw the lips as symmetrical if your lips are uneven. Blend with a complimentary lipstick.
- Add concealer to the outer edges of down-turned lips and add a line to uplift the downward points.

Recommended Makeup Brushes

We recommend you use short handle, natural bristle makeup brushes. The short handle makes it easy to control the makeup application, and they're easy to travel with. Natural bristles are softer and they grab the color better than synthetic bristles. Synthetic bristles can be harsh on your skin, and natural bristle brushes last longer. We recommend you use a brush cleaner, which you can purchase at any beauty supply store. Daily, after using your brushes, you should dip them in the brush cleaner and wipe them on a tissue or a soft cloth. Weekly, you should use a gentle shampoo and cool running water to cleanse your brushes (do not use hot water, as it will damage the bristles). Don't soak your brushes; leave them out to air dry.

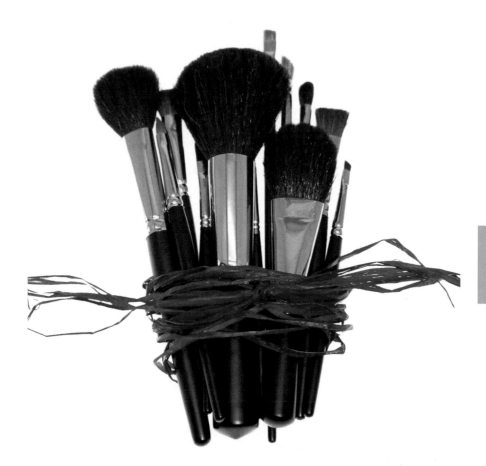

Powder Brush

Super Dome Powder Brush

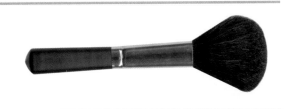

Oversized brush designed to be used after the application of powder foundation to remove excess powder and then again to blend the overall face.

Blush Brushes

Chisel Contour Blush Brush

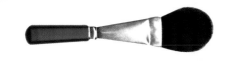

Use to contour and highlight the cheekbone when using a darker blush color.

Chisel Blush Brush

Use to apply the lighter blush color over the darker contour color.

Eyeshadow Brushes

Special Double Shader

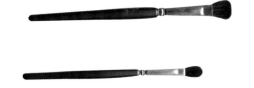

Perfect for applying shadow to the entire eye for a smooth result.

Small Fluff Brush

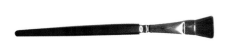

Recommended for the placement of shadow in the hard-to-reach crease of the eye for a more intense, smoky look.

Square Shader #12

This unique shaped brush blends all your color to give a polished yet natural look.

Brow Brushes

Angle Brow

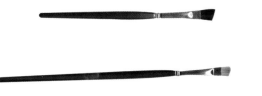

For use with an eyebrow pencil to soften the brow.

Tapered Angle Shader

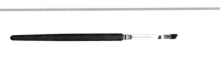

For application of cake brow color.

Eyeliner Brushes

Angle Detailer

This brush is used after using an eyeliner pencil or cake liner to contour and extend the line; also gives a softened line.

Shading Brush

Rounded to a point and designed to be used with a liquid or dry liner.

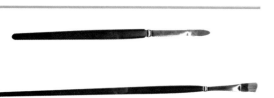

Lip Brushes
Chisel Sable Lip Brush
> The perfect brush for application of lip color after use of your lip liner pencil.
>
> You can also use the Tapered Angle Shader for the application of lip color.

Extras
Good Brush Cleaner

Metal Pencil Sharpener

Makeup Wedges

Duo Fluff/Angle Brush

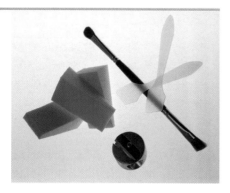

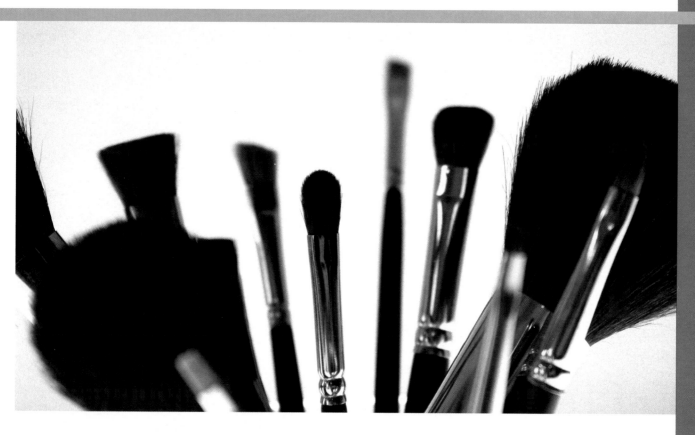

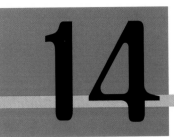# 14 Feng Shui Fashion

Based on the energy of your predominant element, certain choices should be made in the following areas in order to honor you: haircut, hair color, makeup, clothing, accessories, exercise routines, food choices, types of cars, household furniture, garden accessories, people, the best seating arrangement for you, jobs, interview process, etc.; the list is endless! Fashion offers a great opportunity for you to control your image. Simply through your selection of garments, you can manipulate people's impression of you. It's a powerful tool, and I urge my clients to use it.

I recognize that there are circumstances in which your fashion choices may be restricted. Your career may impose practical restraints on the range of your choices. Your budget might discourage you from some options. Even within the restrictions posed by your circumstances, you still have powerful choices. You can use fashion to reinforce your dominant element or you can use it to portray a certain aspect of your personality, an element that may not be fully expressed in your customary style of presenting yourself to the world. By a thoughtful selection of a few key items, you can better present the image that you wish.

When speaking with my clients on this topic, I usually offer the names of well-known designers or clothiers to provide a convenient reference point for a particular style or sensibility. For example, most people will recognize the contrast between the colorful, flamboyant designs of Betsey Johnson and the more classic, understated elegance of Ralph Lauren designs. Similarly, the sophisticated simplicity of Armani designs evokes an entirely different image than the basically wholesome, no-nonsense garments carried by The GAP.

It would be naïve for me to suggest that there's a one-style-fits-all aspect to any of the reference points I provide to my clients and that I've described in this chapter. Of course, each of these designers and clothiers offers garments that are apt to appeal to each of the elements and many of the garments can express different elements just by a slight adjustment in the selection of other garments, shoes, and accessories with which they are worn.

Fashion Tip:
For the ideal blouse neckline, measure from the crown of your head or your hairline to your chin. The deepest neckline you should wear is that same distance, measuring from the chin down to the neckline.

So, how do you select the fashion that's right for you? Or, at least right for the image you're hoping to portray? I'll approach this theme by giving you general guidelines as to the fashion directions that are commonly associated with the each of the five elements. Also, I'll offer you suggestions as to sources for these fashions that are intended to capture a sensibility. Your task is to embrace the suggestions that seem to resonate for you. Forget for a moment the color families. If you are a fire personality, I do not expect to see you only in reds and purples! Rather, I want you to think in terms of the energy of the clothing.

Fire

Fire shines. It is alive and spirited. Fire personalities are spirited, enthusiastic, risk-taking, charismatic, and passionate. When I think of my Fire clientele, they are often the first to wear the latest designs. These individuals are quick to look for expressive ways to define their creative self and are less likely to be bound by tradition or formality. Clothing for Fire types should reflect their creative nature. Fire types aren't shy about mixing retro fashion with a modern piece of clothing for an expressive, unique look, and might add a pair of Jimmy Choo shoes to complete the outfit.

Clothing for Fire types that feels alive, nonrestrictive, and vibrant is best. The Fire types are drawn to clothing that not only says, "Wow!" but also allows the magnetic personality of the wearer to shine. Working in platform boots while sporting the latest Palazzo pantsuit doesn't faze Fire types. If the clothing is fun and makes a statement, it is all the better. Accessories are larger than life or totally bold and unique in color and design.

To be clear, too much Fire or Fire out of control can take what would otherwise be a daringly beautiful fashion statement and turn it into a clown suit, so use suitable discretion. Even if your circumstances require you to honor a conservative dress code for your career, you can express your Fire element in simple but expressive ways. For example, some of my male clients are required to wear a suit and tie every day, so they'll often select a more spirited, bold tie as their statement. For some, the selection of a distinctive piece of jewelry will provide the keynote of individuality and expressiveness.

Designers/Sources for Fire
Versace
Betsey Johnson
Dolce & Gabana
Christian Dior

Earth

Earth supports. It is solid and fertile. Earth personalities are nurturing, down-to-earth, centered, and calm. Many of my Earth clients dress nicely but would rather the focus not be on their clothing. Their clothing often is practical and may be mixed with a smorgasbord of other articles. Clothing that appeals to Earth types will not draw attention to them, but rather serves as either comfort clothing or merely serves the utilitarian function of covering up.

At the risk of leading you to believe that Earth types don't take pride in their style, please know that my experience has shown that earth clients would rather the message be found in their actions rather than their garments. Clothing that supports that message is usually practical and comfortable, such as cotton or linen suits. Typically, simple, unfettered lines and practical, wearable fabrics are the hallmarks of Earth style.

Designers/Sources for Earth
Ellen Tracy
J. Jill
Eileen Fisher
Liz Claiborne

Metal

Metal reinforces. It is perfection and order. It is clean lines and no-fuss details. Reliable, traditional, efficient, dependable clothing, classic traditional lines that are timeless; these are the hallmarks of Metal style. Clothing that says right up front, "I mean business." My Metal clientele wear classic clothing even on Saturdays! On the tennis court or golf course, they are impeccably dressed. Even to the casual observer, it's apparent that Metal types pay keen attention to the details of their attire. You may find your Metal husband pulling weeds in his Cole Haan shoes.

A Metal type would never go out in public without flawless makeup, hair, and clothing. A Metal type will keep a classic purse or piece of clothing for a long time as the lines are timeless. My Metal clients often speak to me in amazement at the casual dress they find in the courtroom, the church, at school, etc. Flamboyant, alternative, and anything that resembles sloppiness, are contrary to the Metal style. Metal style finds a way to make even an older pair of Levis look orderly.

Designers/Sources for Metal
Hugo Boss
Brooks Brothers
Chanel
Giorgio Armani

Water

Water flows. It refreshes and restores. Water types are visionaries, chic while thoughtful and reflective. Their style sense tends toward clothing that offers fashion without restriction, sensual clothing that offers balance in design. My Water clients often will be wearing the most fashionable clothing. Compared to Fire types, Water style tends towards fashionable choices that are likely to stay in style for a while, not fade away after one or two seasons. Their clothing choices are smart yet forward-looking. I find my Water clients are the most open to change. Water clients have a flirty, but not necessarily seductive, approach to dress. Water style is most represented by a chic elegance.

Designers/Sources for Water
Donna Karan
Calvin Klein
Prada
Carolina Herrera

Wood

Wood springs. It is strong and flexible. Wood types are on the go and are usually competitive. Many of my wood clientele are athletic to some degree; however, even if not involved in any sport, Wood types are movers. Their clothing, whether professional or personal, must not restrict. They must not be hindered by their clothing. Their clothing must enable them to do (operative word, "do") whatever they want to accomplish. As most Wood types are go-getters, the clothing must be part of the approach. In their design, the clothing must support the effort. For more formal fashion, Wood style often suggests a level of power, strength, or success. On the casual side, Wood fashion is more connected to the active lifestyles of the Wood element.

Designers/Sources for Wood
Ralph Lauren Polo
Banana Republic
DKNY
J.Crew

These suggestions aren't intended as an all-inclusive, final authority, closed list. Instead, they're offered as a suggestion of some of the sources that are most likely to appeal to the specific element types. These suggestions are intended as a weather vane to point out the spirit of these elements in terms of fashion. Like most of what you'll find in this book, you should embrace the recommendations that are comfortable for you and adapt a plan that best expresses your individuality.

15 Yamaguchi Hair Therapy

Yamaguchi Feng Shui Make-over

What a fantastic opportunity awaits me each day as I prepare for the work day. I feel as though I am an artist waiting for the canvas to tell me what to paint. In my case, it is the guest who shares with me who she is and what she does. After an in-depth consultation and exchange of information, the guest and I identify the dominant element in her life. We look at the yin/yang energy within the element. Does she have too much of the dominant element? If so, I need to reduce it by balancing the element. If her appearance does not reflect her element, I need to enhance it or add more of the element. If she is just slightly out of balance, I can harmonize it by introducing other elements.

It isn't just a cut, color, or makeup that we offer. It is the whole Feng Shui experience that allows us to make a difference in the guest's appearance and life. It gives the guest the opportunity to participate in sound decisions based on her answers. We can take sacred steps to reach the guest's goal or we can make visible changes in one appointment. It depends upon the guest. We believe in honoring the guest by listening to her and by recommending changes that are in keeping with her element.

The changes you see in the following case studies may be subtle or startling; however, all of the changes are not obvious. We make recommendations for new opportunities and growth in their lives. I am grateful for my guests who have allowed me to share in their lives.

Fire

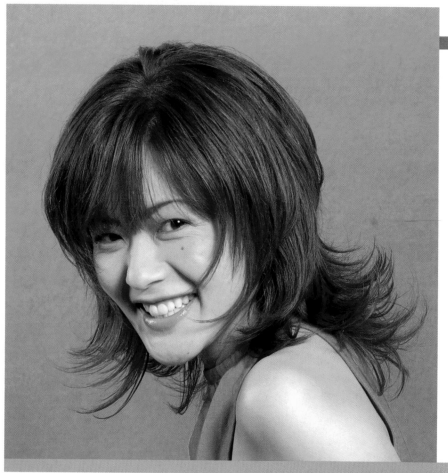

Sayaka

Face Shape: Round
Skin Tone: Honey
Elements: Fire/Earth

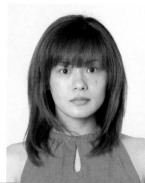

Sayaka is very expressive and artistic. When she came in, her look did not reflect the spark and energy that defines her. I wanted to create a bold haircut that would enhance her Fire element. She wanted to keep her hair long, so in the Fire hair cut I created bold disconnected pieces for an expressive style. Her deep cinnamon hair color matches her red-brown eyes. To harmonize the Fire element and to enhance the Earth element, soft Earth makeup completed her new look.

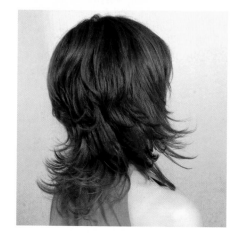

Sachi

Face Shape: Heart
Skin Tone: Olive
Elements: Fire/Wood

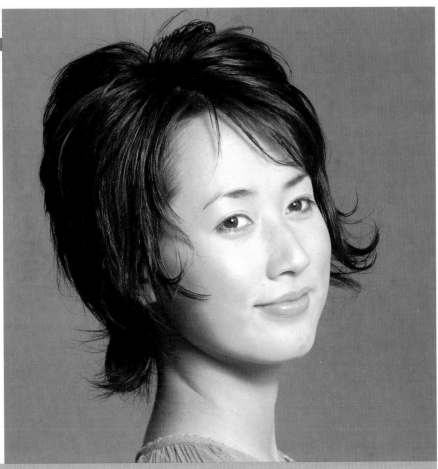

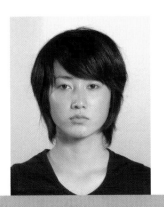

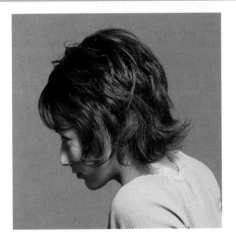

Sachi is very artistic and passionate about life. When she came into the salon her look was Earth—a no fuss style. I enhanced the Fire with her cut that is disconnected with uneven pieces. Since her face is heart shape, I wanted to have longer pieces that flip out at the jawline to add width for balance. The Fire highlights have random pieces of red throughout her dark brown hair. I harmonized her makeup with Wood to keep a soft muted look.

Fire

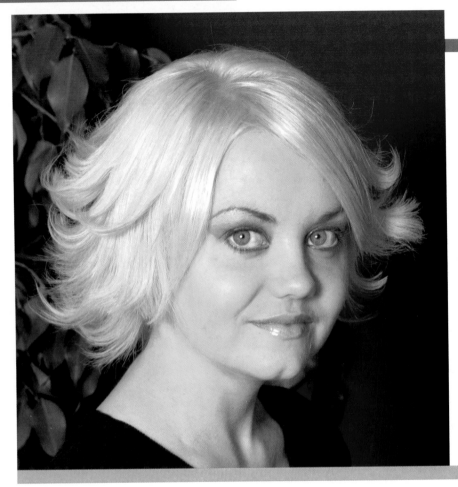

Lizzy

Face Shape: Heart
Skin Tone: Porcelain
Elements: Fire/Water

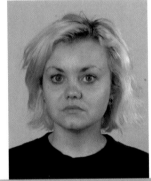

Lizzy's profession and her hobbies provide a venue for her artistic talents. She is a photographer as well as a musician. She plays bass guitar for a rockabilly band. I wanted to keep a look that was expressive, artistic, and one that would serve her well on stage. Her cut is very expressive, disconnected, and alternative. She is very artistic and confident so she is able to wear a Fire haircut, color, and makeup.

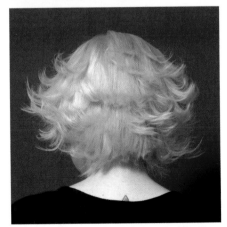

Sara

Face Shape: Round
Skin Tone: Porcelain
Elements: Fire/Wood

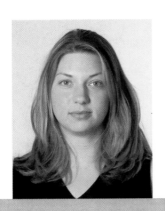

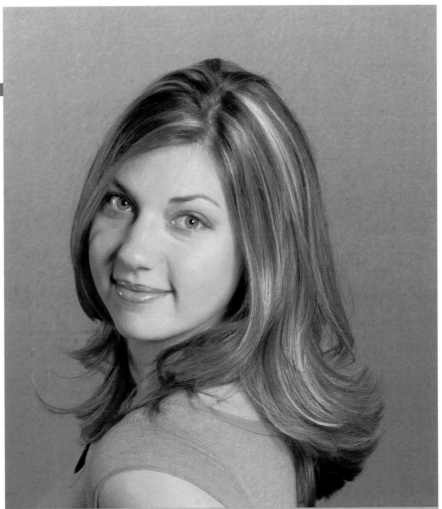

Sara made a career change with the birth of her baby and became a full time stay-at-home mom. She still needed an expression for her artistic talent as a writer. Her personality is very expressive and people are aware of her presence. Her hair was kept long with a Wood haircut that added movement. The Fire color and highlights added the spark and energy that reflected Sara's enthusiasm. Wood makeup added the subtle touch for her porcelain skin.

Earth

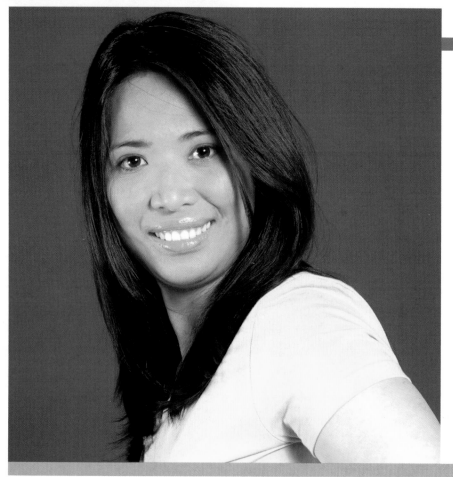

Denise

Face Shape: Oval
Skin Tone: Honey
Elements: Earth/Metal

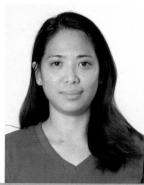

When Denise came into the salon she had a very easy, no-fuss hair style. Her warm personality and love for people was obvious from the first encounter. Although she spends more time caring for others than herself, I enhanced the Earth element to create a soft look by cutting round layers around her face. Her Earth haircut, color, and makeup project a calm demeanor that is important to her career. Her position as a medical caregiver requires her to be nurturing as well as precise and organized.

Ally

Face Shape: Oval
Skin Tone: Milky
Elements: Earth/Fire

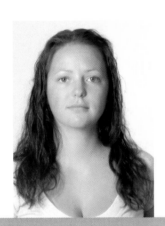

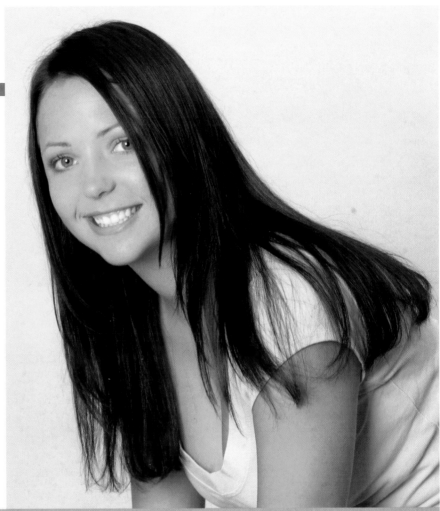

Ally returned home from an exciting two months in Paris, France, where she has decided to spend the year as a live-in nanny for triplets. Her nurturing personality along with her newly chosen career was the determining factor for enhancing the Earth element. Her Earth haircut offers her the freedom to wear many styles. A rich auburn hair color enhances her beautiful skin. Her soft Earth makeup showcases her eyes and smile.

Earth

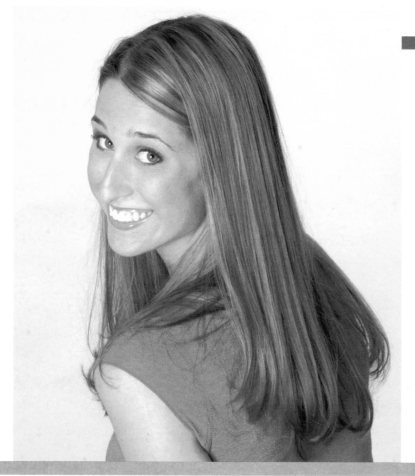

Katie

Face Shape: Oblong
Skin Tone: Milky
Elements: Earth/Wood

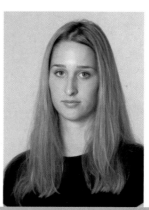

Katie is very social and, like most teenagers, loves to be around her friends. She described herself as intuitive, caring, and nurturing with her friends and family. She loves to play tennis and basketball. Her active life requires a style that takes little time but that reflects her inner beauty. She wanted to keep her hair long as it offers a variety of styling possibilities. Her Earth highlights are very natural and sun-kissed. Earth makeup enhances already perfect skin.

Mikella

Face Shape: Oblong
Skin Tone: Honey
Elements: Earth/Wood

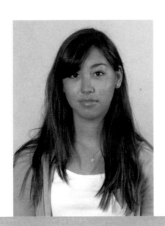

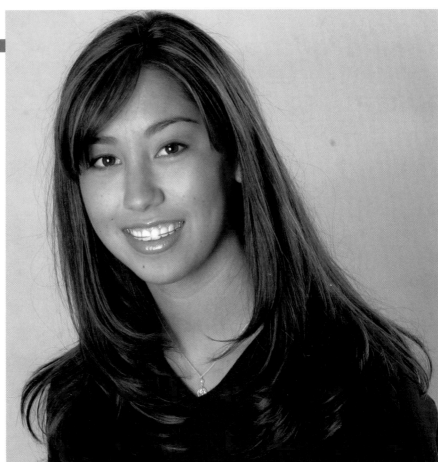

Mikella is very active in school and various outside activities. She prefers to spend very little time on her hair. She wanted to keep the length of her hair. We softened the colors around her face with Earth colors and highlights. The Earth cut has soft movement and offers a variety of ways to style her hair. She wears very little makeup and was receptive to subtle Earth colors which look very natural.

Metal

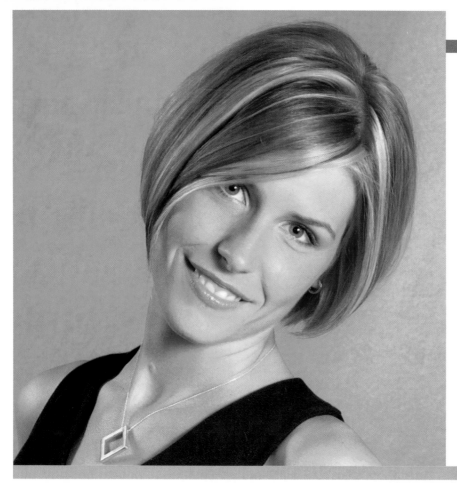

Amy

Face Shape: Oval
Skin Tone: Milky
Elements: Metal/Fire

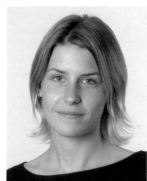

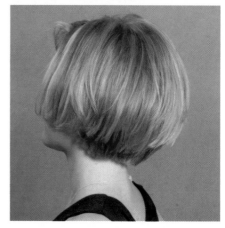

Amy is extremely organized and disciplined concerning her career. She is daring and always seeking a change or new adventure. She just returned from five months in Spain and was ready to pursue her goals. Her desire is to manage a spa and/or salon and she needed a professional style. Her haircut is Metal in its sleek, classic style, while her hair color and highlights are definitely Fire. She was hired as a spa director shortly after the make-over.

Heather

Face Shape: Oval
Skin Tone: Milky
Elements: Metal/Fire

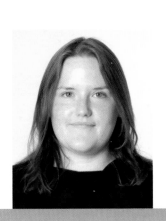

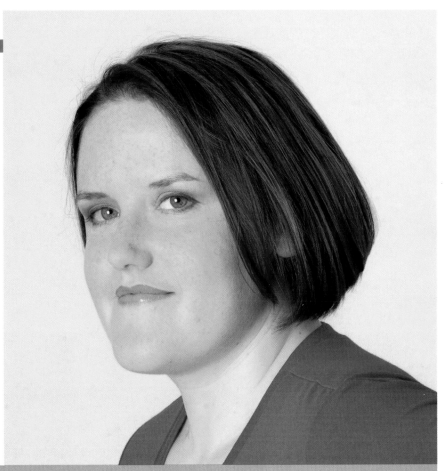

Heather's new management position with a theatre company puts her in the best of both worlds. Her position requires her to be focused and organized. She describes herself as artistic and adventurous as well as disciplined. A Metal hair cut gives a sleek, professional appearance. Her hair color was darkened and Metal highlights add depth to the color and make the hair appear thicker. She doesn't usually wear makeup so soft Earth colors were applied to harmonize the Metal element.

Metal

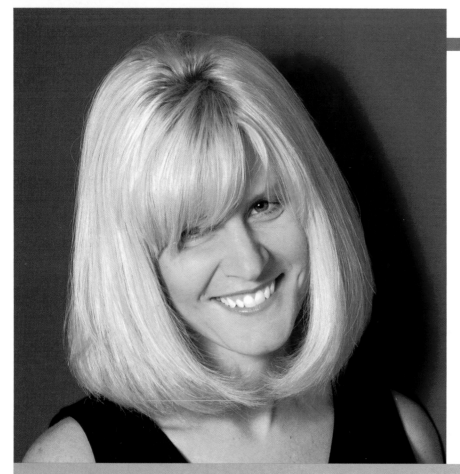

Norma

Face Shape: Oval
Skin Tone: Porcelain
Elements: Metal/Metal

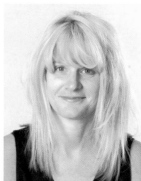

Norma's position as the director of production for a publishing company requires that she have a professional appearance. She is disciplined, organized, and extremely efficient in her work and in her personal life. After our consultation, I let Norma know that it would take sacred steps to take her hair where she wanted it to be. When moisture is taken from the hair with bleaching, deep conditioning is required at least weekly to replenish the hair. I wanted to enhance her Metal element by giving her a one length bob. Cool blonde was added to the color to tone down the gold. She wanted to keep long bangs; my next goal is to have the bangs grow out to show her face and blue eyes.

Heidi

Face Shape: Square
Skin Tone: Porcelain
Elements: Metal/Wood

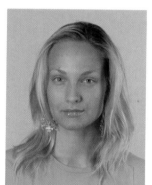

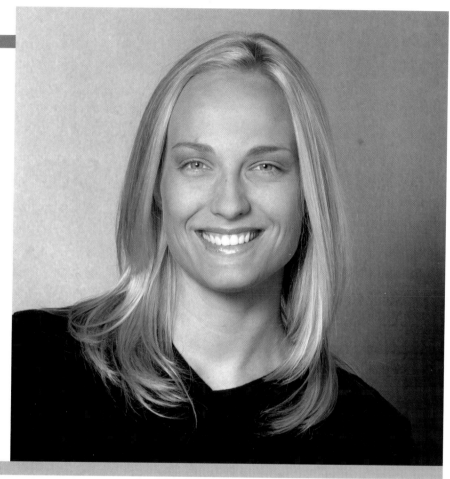

Heidi has an interesting career as a fashion stylist. It is her organizational skills and precise attention to details that make her in demand for photo shoots and television. She is very social and loves being with others. She is focused and disciplined about her exercise regimen. I chose to enhance the Metal element which balances Wood. She wanted a change that reflects her professional status but that was not too rigid. Her hair cut is sleek with long, soft-cut lines that frame her face. I added cool blonde highlights to enhance her blue eyes and porcelain skin. Her Wood makeup is both soft and classic.

Water

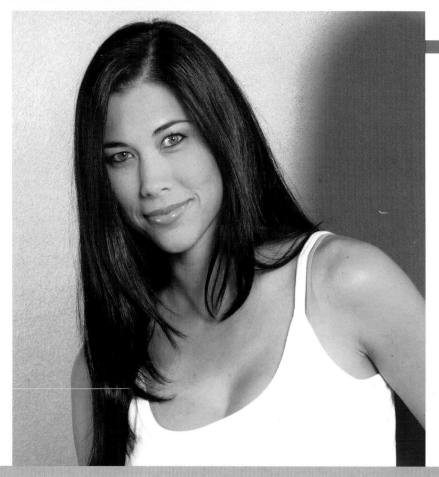

Sarah

Face Shape: Oval
Skin Tone: Honey
Elements: Water/Wood

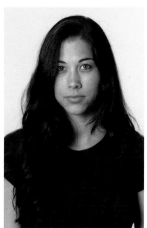

Sarah is a makeup artist who wanted to reflect a chic image. She is extremely social and enjoys great rapport with her clients. She is a single mom on the go and wanted a professional appearance that would also adapt to her busy life style. She practices yoga and Pilates daily. The hair cut was trimmed to one length with long soft layers framing her neckline. One color was applied to her hair to eliminate the different colors from previous coloring applications. Water makeup accentuates her beautiful almond eyes for the finishing touches to a chic, sensual look.

Hayley

Face Shape: Square
Skin Tone: Porcelain
Elements: Water/Fire

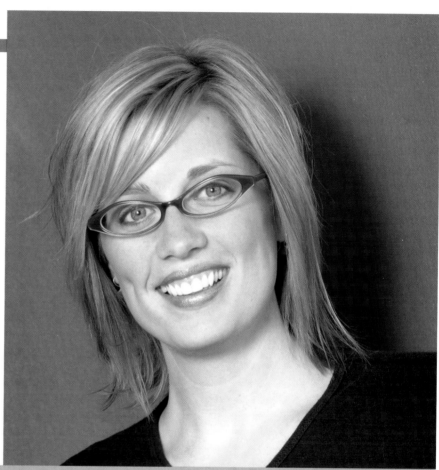

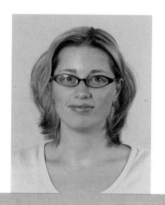

Hayley stated that she loves life and works so that she can enjoy it. She enjoys traveling and outdoor activities such as scuba diving. Her love for adventure and willingness to try something new is tempered only by her desire to be cautious and have full information before starting the journey. I added cool blonde colors with Water highlights to bring out the blue in her eyes. The Water haircut provides a look both professional and chic. Water makeup enhanced her beautiful porcelain skin and completed the make-over.

Water

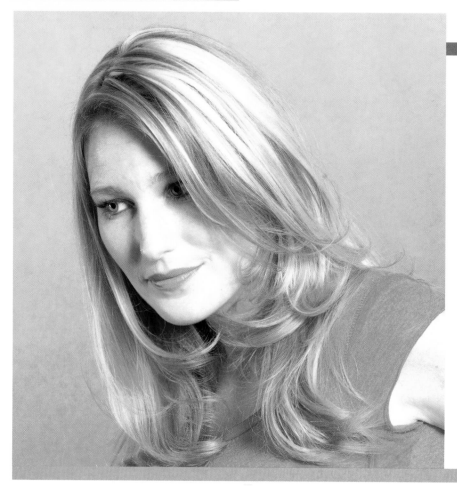

Ashlee

Face Shape: Oblong
Skin Tone: Porcelain
Elements: Water/Earth

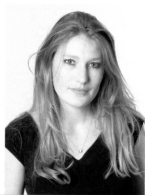

Ashlee's love of reading and quiet time for herself is blended with her career as a spa esthetician. Her quiet, nurturing demeanor endears her to her clients and co-workers. She wanted a professional appearance to match her new career. With her vertical body type, I kept her hair long and horizontal with flirty kicks around her face. To go along with the Water cut, I added cooler highlights using a Water pattern. Water makeup completed her chic, professional make-over.

Sammie

Face Shape: Oval
Skin Tone: Porcelain
Elements: Water/Fire

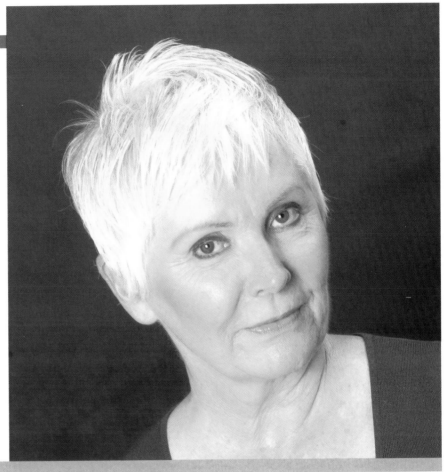

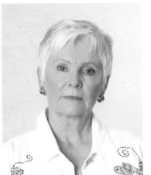

When Sammie first came into the salon, she was wearing a Metal bob hair cut. During the consultation, I discovered that I would need to take sacred steps to achieve the look that reflected Sammie's elements. Her profession as an administrator required a professional appearance, however, it did not require a severe one as she is very social. I wanted to make her more chic and not so restricted. During the second appointment, I added texture for a more chic, sassy appearance. I controlled the yellow in her hair and added violet to achieve the cool color that showcases her blue eyes. Her Water makeup added the finishing touch.

Wood

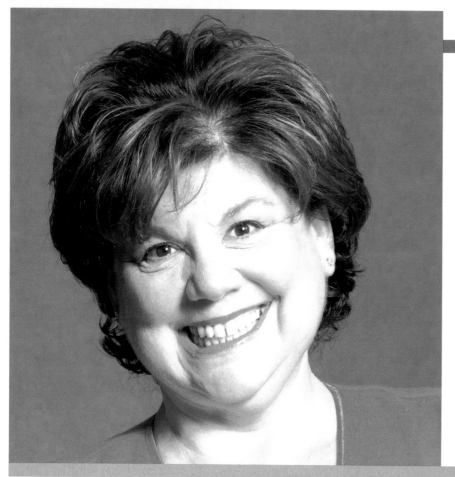

Lois

Face Shape: Round
Skin Tone: Milky
Elements: Wood/Fire

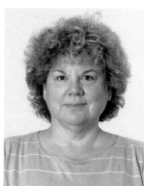

Lois is a closet Fire masquerading as a bookkeeper. She is artistic, fun, and loves to travel. She is very outgoing and has an effervescent personality. When Lois first sat in my chair, she had an Earth appearance. I knew that she was hiding the beauty inside. I harmonized the Fire element and enhanced the Wood element by giving her a professional, yet youthful, appearance. The deep cinnamon hair color enhanced her milky skin and matched her red-brown eyes. I added Wood highlights to lengthen her face shape. I created a controlled, tousled haircut. With soft Wood makeup, we had achieved a make-over that she said fit her exactly.

Sara

Face Shape: Oval
Skin Tone: Milky
Elements: Wood/Water

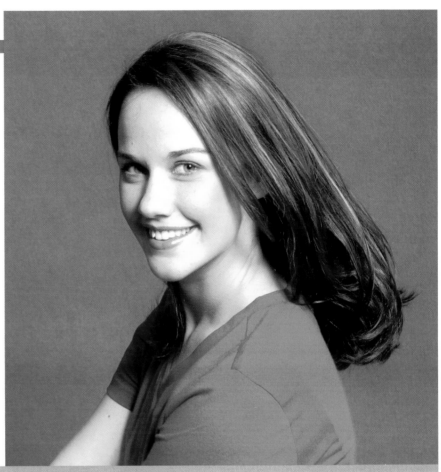

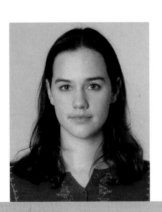

Sara loves being around people, being in the limelight, and participating in activities. She is outgoing and enjoys the attention of others. By reading and finding time for herself, she finds a balance in her busy life as an actress and drama student. Her appearance was very casual, no-fuss, reflecting Earth element. The Wood haircut was left long to give her a variety of styling options. I added long layers for movement and Wood highlights in a caramel color to add texture to her dark, rich brown hair. Water makeup was added for a chic look.

Wood

Dawn

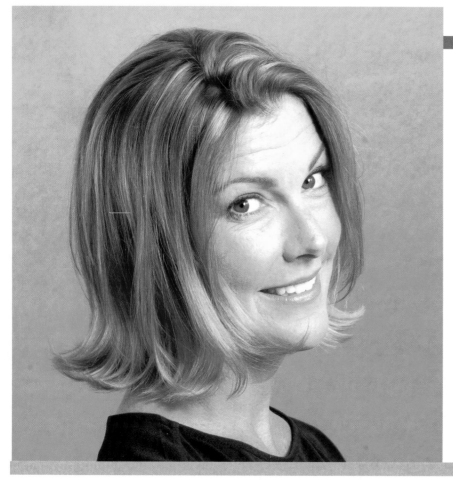

Face Shape: Oval
Skin Tone: Milky
Elements: Wood/Fire

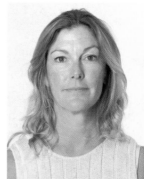

Dawn loves being involved with the outdoors. She is very active and enjoys the ocean and running. She wanted a more professional appearance as well as one that allowed her to be involved in her outside activities. I cut her hair at her perfect length and added texture. The Wood colors and highlights created a more youthful appearance. The soft Wood makeup completed the make-over.

Megan

Face Shape: Oblong
Skin Tone: Milky
Elements: Wood/Metal

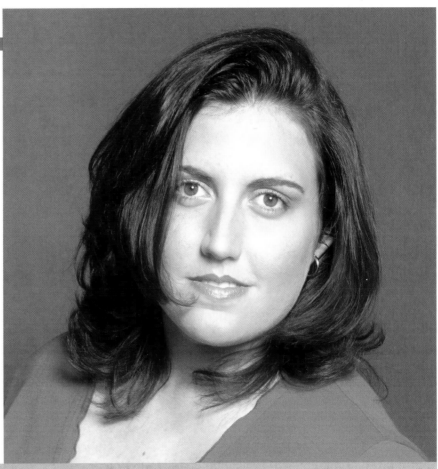

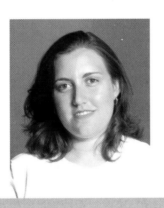

When Megan first sat in my chair, her appearance was more of a college student than a professional graphic designer. She leads an active life that leaves her little time to fret about her hair. I enhanced her Wood element by texturizing the hair for volume and movement. I placed the first layer at the jaw line to shorten her oblong face. Her rich, chocolate-brown hair showcases her milky skin and dark eyes. Subtle, muted makeup completes the look for an active professional.

Tips and Techniques

I'm pleased to share with you lots of tips and techniques for your hair; brushing, combing, shampooing, conditioning, and styling. At the end of this chapter you'll find a listing of products that I've developed over years of working with hair and skin.

Combing and Brushing

- Don't brush or comb your hair before shampooing. Plan to get the tangles out after you've conditioned.
- Brush the scalp with a bristle brush to exfoliate the scalp and to aid circulation.
- For medium to fine hair, use a fine-toothed comb.
- For medium to thick hair, use a wide-toothed comb.
- If your hair is naturally curly, use a moisturizing leave-in conditioner and use a pick to detangle the hair. Once or twice a week, use a deep conditioner.
- For medium to fine straight hair, use a metal brush to blow-dry because the bristles will get hot and curl the hair.
- For medium to fine straight hair, use a boar bristle brush to blow-dry to achieve a sleek, smooth style.
- For naturally curly to wavy hair, use a boar bristle brush for blow-drying because it will help straighten the hair and flatten the cuticle, giving your style more shine.
- For curly hair, apply a gel-type product, not a mousse, and dry it with a diffuser.
- For short hair, use a brush with plastic tips on the bristles for blow-drying, as it grabs the hair and gives you more control as you style.

Shampooing and Conditioning

- If your hair is oily, don't use hot water. Use tepid to warm water, although cool is even better. Shampoo without rubbing the scalp, because rubbing stimulates the sebaceous glands and increases oils.
- For normal scalp, wash with warm water then rinse with cold water to seal off the cuticle and give your hair shine.
- If you have color-treated hair, use a product without detergents. If you can't, wash with warm water and rinse in cold. This will keep the color in longer.
- People with long hair (below the breastbone) should shampoo every two to three days.
- All types of hair, with the exception of really fine hair, should be conditioned daily, or at least every other day. (Fine hair will flatten with this much conditioning.)
- Naturally curly hair's best friend is a deep conditioner. Comb conditioner through the hair. If you don't, conditioner stays on the hump of the curl and it should be evenly distributed in the concave as well. The ends are always the driest on curly hair.

Color

- If you are on a budget, highlight in the part and only recolor the base.
- If you're blonde and the sun lightens your hair too much, add some lowlights for contrast.
- Don't shampoo the day following the application of color. Let the color set for a day.

Styling

- Thick hair may hold moisture, so use a Japanese sponge or chamois towel until 50 percent of the moisture is out of the hair. Then style.
- If you're going to use a blow-dryer, get one that blows hard, as it dries hotter. The less time blow-drying the hair the better it is for the hair.
- If your blow-dryer comes with a funnel, do not throw it away as funnels direct the heat where it needs to go.
- If a blow-dryer does not come with a diffuser make sure that it's a standard cylinder for adding a separate diffuser.
- If you have a difficult time styling medium to fine hair with a blow-dryer, I recommend using hot rollers after your hair is completely dry.
- If your hair is thick, use a brush for blow-drying, or a flat iron for straight, sleek hair.
- To create a tighter curl with a curling iron, start from the base of the strand of hair and curl to the ends. Feed the ends of the hair into the barrel last. For a looser curl, start from the ends and curl up.
- Gold curling irons get hottest. Silver curling irons offer less heat.
- The larger the barrel of the curling iron, the softer the curl will be and the more movement the curl will have. The smaller the barrel, the tighter and more long lasting the curl will be. Hair should wrap around the barrel at least twice to get the true size of the curl.
- If you want a crisp curl in your medium to fine hair, use an aerosol or pump hair spray and spray each section of hair prior to wrapping it around the curling iron barrel.
- For styling naturally curly hair, after blow-drying or curling lean your head all the way forward and tousle the hair with your hands from roots to ends, then throw your head up and toss the hair back. With your fingertips, arrange the curls in a more uniform balance.
- For straight to wavy hair, do the same thing except at the end, use your hands with your fingers spread, tousling the hair so it spreads the hair out.
- If your hair is overly fine, be careful when teasing. Make sure the hair is well conditioned.

Applying Products

- Rub add-in or finishing hair products over both sides of the hands. You'll get better distribution of the product as you go through the hair.
- Apply product starting from the middle or the inside, then go underneath. Product will then support the mass of the hair.

Hair Loss

- Birth control pills, other types of medication, menopause, poor diet, and a deficiency of enzymes and minerals can cause hair loss. If you feel you are losing too much hair, speak with your doctor.
- The five top causes for hair loss are:
    1. Medication
    2. Excessive changing of diet
    3. Hereditary
    4. Stress
    5. Menopause
- Possible solutions to hair loss include:
    1. Supplements
    2. Beta Carotene
    3. B12, B6, B complex
    4. Zinc
    5. Scalp massage
- Make sure you're not using products that clog follicles

Yamaguchi Hair Therapy Products

Yamaguchi Hair Therapy products were created out of our frustration with inferior products on the market. We use only pure botanical extracts and essential oils because we want to provide our clients with the most effective and highest quality products available.

Based on your dominant element, choose among these products:

Fire	Earth	Metal	Water	Wood
Soy shampoo	Soy shampoo	Soy shampoo	Soy shampoo	Soy shampoo
Watercress conditioner	Watercress conditioner	Watercress conditioner	Watercress conditioner	Watercress conditioner
Shine	Shine		Shine	Shine
	Silk	Silk	Silk	Silk
Full Spray Mousse	Green Tea Shape	Full Spray Mousse	Full Spray Mousse	Full Spray Mousse
Green Tea Shape	Smoothing Balm	Green Tea Shape	Green Tea Shape	Green Tea Shape
Herbal Gel	Polish	Herbal Gel	Herbal Gel	Herbal Gel
Sake Hairspray		Sake Hairspray	Smoothing Balm	Smoothing Balm
Smoothing Balm		Polish	Polish	Polish
Polish			Rice Putty	Rice Putty
Rice Putty				
Bamboo Paste	Bamboo Paste	Bamboo Paste	Bamboo Paste	Bamboo Paste

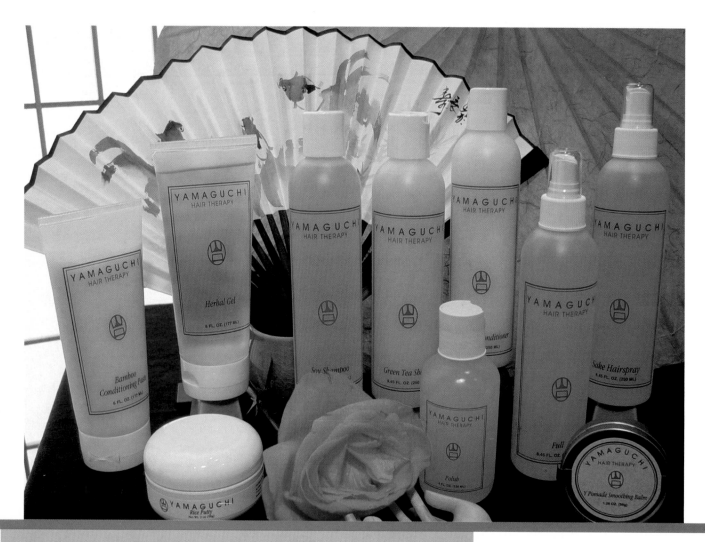

Yamaguchi Hair Therapy Products

For more information or to order any of our products, please visit our website at www.yamaguchifengshui.com.

Bamboo Conditioning Paste
Whole leaf aloe vera, whole wheat protein, bamboo extracts, and lavender oil plus Simethicone. Replenish environmentally and chemically damaged hair.

Herbal Gel
Whole leaf aloe vera for luster and control. A natural sunscreen and a must for curly hair.

Soy Shampoo
Soy derivatives provide the sudsing agent. Locks in color.

Green Tea Shape
Moisturizing green tea extracts allow natural styling without stiffness. Alcohol free.

Silk Leave-In Conditioner
Silk protein detangles hair and eliminates static electricity.

Watercress Conditioner
Silk protein blended with whole wheat protein protects and adds luster while moisturizing and nourishing the hair.

Sake Hairspray
Non-drying sake derivatives provide exceptional hold without drying.

Rice Putty
Whole leaf aloe vera concentrate, hydrogenated lanolin, squalene, rice bran oil. Separates hair as desired for curly or textured looks.

Polish
Aloe oil and herbal extracts moisturize and eliminate frizz. Creates smooth, shiny, silky hair while providing a natural sunscreen. Add to Watercress Conditioner for detangling and mix with Green Tea Shape for a great hold.

Full Spray Mousse
Aloe vera, kiwi extract in this great volumizer. Wonderful for curly and fine hair.

Pomade Smoothing Balm
Shea butter and beeswax ease frizz to create a sleek, smooth finish. Accents shorter, angular cuts.

Shine
Carrot, wheat germ, and borage oils create sheen while controlling hair. Spray all over for a great shine. A natural sunscreen.

Our Yamaguchi Spa Therapy Feng Shui Essential Oil features five distinct themes, each theme offering distinct benefits and linked to the five elements of Feng Shui: Fire, Earth, Metal, Water, and Wood.

FIRE/harmony: A union of eucalyptus, Siberian fir, sandalwood, and mint
EARTH/serenity: A mixture of lavender, chamomile, marjoram, and sandalwood
METAL/signature: A tender fusion of citrus notes, florals, woods, and vanilla
WATER/tranquility: A blend of lavender, rose, cardamom, and geranium
WOOD/balance: A blend of spearmint, balsamic rosemary, bay, and lavender

Each product within the Feng Shui Line is available in each of these five themes.

Sealers
Replenishes skin with fifteen aromatic flower and herb essences to hydrate and nourish skin. Vitamins A, E, and jojoba oil refresh, sooth, and tone the skin and hair. Seals in moisture.

Cleanser
Ideal for the entire body, including the hair. Herbal extracts and flower essences naturally control odor and bacteria.

Scrub
Finely milled loofah and crushed apricot seeds exfoliate surface impurities without drying. Replenishes natural oils.

Emollient Balm
Protects skin from the environment. Enriched with Vitamin A, C, and D and macadamia nut oil to preserve a healthy youthful skin.

Oils
Aromatherapy blended from nature's pure essential oils into a rich jojoba, evening primrose, and borage oil base. Great for hair, skin, and nail care.

Salts
Detoxifying sea salts enriched with sea kelp nourish, condition, and soften the skin.

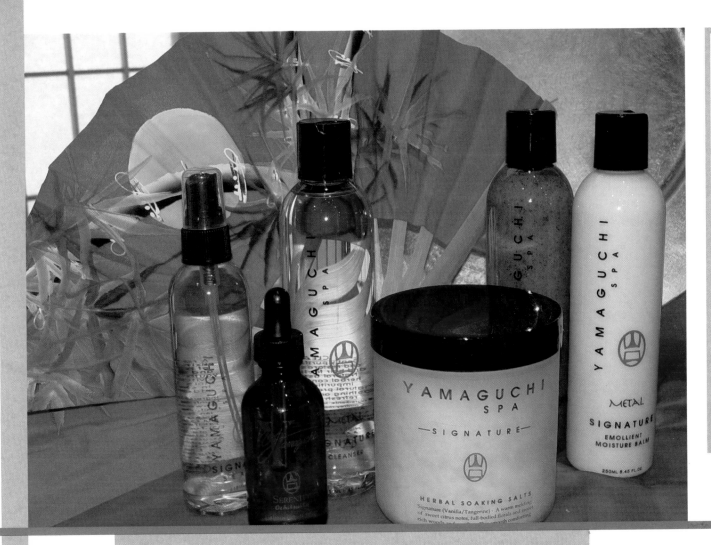

Yamaguchi Feng Shui Spa Products

For more information or to order any of our products, please visit our website at www.yamaguchifengshui.com.

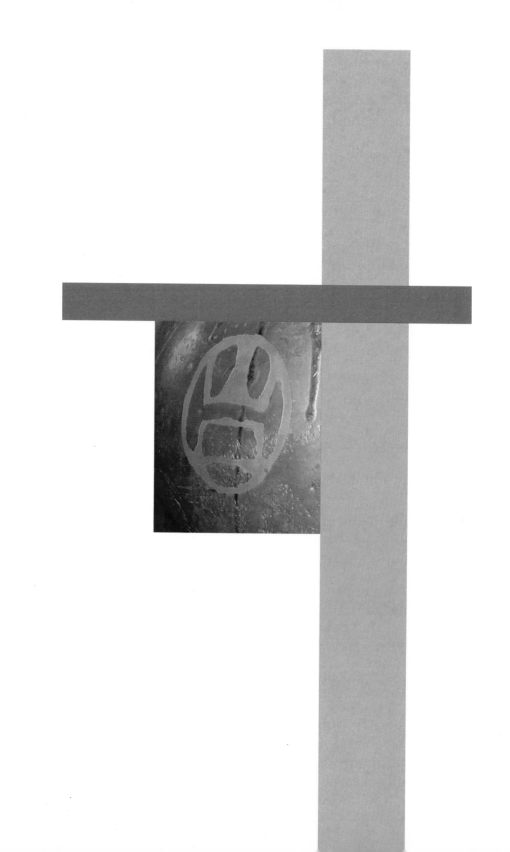

Appendix Hair Coloring Techniques for Stylists

Yamaguchi Feng Shui Foundation

This foundation creates a common language, provides specific instruction to team members, prevents product waste, and guarantees consistency.

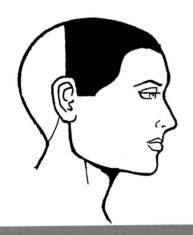

Reference Points

- Pivot of the head
- Top of the ears
- Outer corners of the eyes
- Occipital bone
- Curvature of the head

Divisions

Division A

- The reference point is from the top of the left ear to the top of the right ear.
- Everything forward is Division A.

Division B

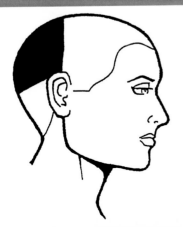

- The top reference point is from the top of the left ear to the top of the right ear. The bottom reference point is from the top of the left ear to the occipital bone and from the top of the right ear to the occipital bone.
- Everything between is Division B.

Division C

- Everything below Division B is Division C.

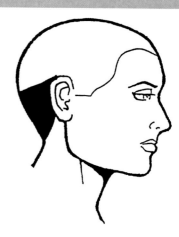

Panels
Horizontal

- The reference points are from the outer left eye following the curvature of the head to the occipital bone and the outer right eye following the curvature of the head to the occipital bone. Everything above is the Horizontal Panel.

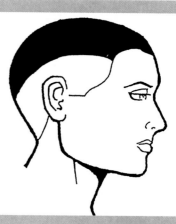

Vertical

- Everything below the Horizontal Panel is the Vertical Panel.

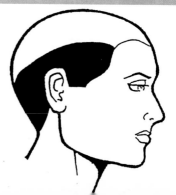

Detail Panels

Quarter Panel—HP ¼

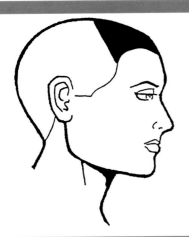

- The Quarter Panel is from the outer left eye to half the distance of the pivot of the head to the hair line, and from the outer right eye to half the distance of the pivot of the head.

One Half Panel—HP ½

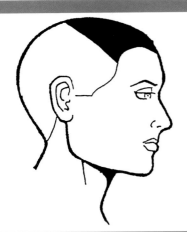

- The One Half Panel is from the outer left eye to the pivot of the head and from the outer right eye to the pivot of the head.

Three Quarter Panel—HP ¾

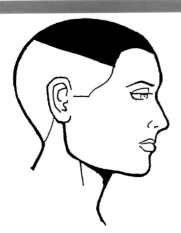

- The Three Quarter Panel is from the corner of the outer left eye following the curvature of the head to half the distance from pivot of the head to the occipital bone and from the outer corner of the right eye following the curvature of the head to half the distance from the pivot of the head to the occipital bone.

Division A in the Vertical Panel—AV

- Division A in the Vertical Panel is from the outer point of the eye following the curvature of the head down to the top of the left ear or the top of the right ear.

Yamaguchi Feng Shui Color Techniques

Element	Fire	Earth	Metal	Water	Wood
Color	Artistic	Natural	Elegant classic	Elegant chic	Sporty
Techniques	Slice, Tokyo highlights	4-6 pieces weave	7-9 pieces weave	2-7 pieces weave	4-4 pieces weave
	2-4 colors used	2-4 colors used	1-2-3 colors used	1-2-3 colors used	2-3 colors used
	Anything goes in level range	2 up 2 down level range	4 up 3 down level range	5 up 4 down level range	3 up 2 down level range

Heart

Wide forehead, face draws to a point at chin.

1. Place darker color on the outer corner of fringes (bangs).

2. In the back of Division A, begin highlights toward center of forehead to draw attention up.

3. Side-swept fringes look great, but they must hit at cheek level. You can highlight.

4. Bottom flip—add highlights to Division C hairline.

5. Make AV panel darker, but Division C area lighter.

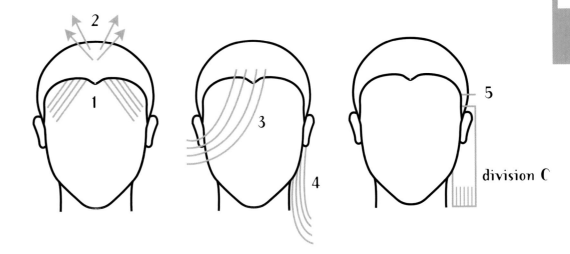

division C

Oval

1. This is the ideal face shape.

2. Keep ¼ of an inch around the entire hairline solid so the face shape will not change.

3. Color and highlight according to skin tone, eye tone, and haircut style. Stay off the hairline ¼ an inch around.

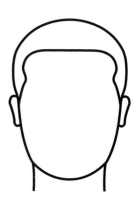

Face is round but slightly elongated, jaw is as wide as forehead.

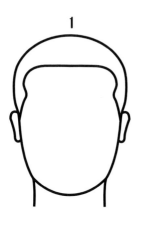

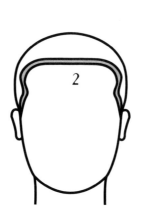

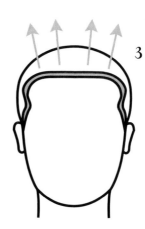

Round

1. Part down the middle and smooth fringes to the side. Keep Division A ¼ HP dark.

2. Add highlights to top area to create height.

3. On an off-set part, add highlights to back of Division A.

4. Keep Division AV panel darker to slenderize face.

5. Long hair and all hair styles that frame the face need to have darker colors for depth.

6. Bobs that are cut to the lip need to be darker toward the bottom.

Face looks full and wide, distance between the lower lip and end of the chin is short.

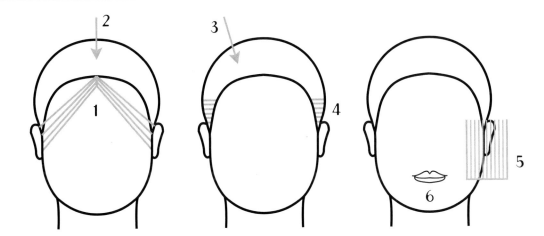

Square

1. On fringes, the outside corners need to be darker or solid.

2. Middle parts slim the width of square faces.

3. Add highlights toward the center of the head to draw focal point away from width.

4. Create side-swept fringe ending at the cheek area to add softness to the jaw.

5. With medium to long lengths, keep the vertical panel darker or untouched with highlights.

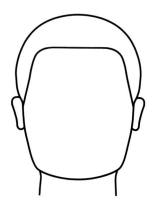

Strong, angular jawline and wide forehead.

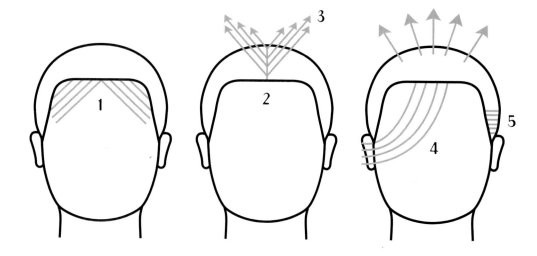

Oblong

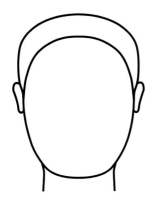

Equal in width from forehead to jawline, with a more linear appearance than an oval shaped face.

1. Fringes on the face need to be darker to shorten the face shape.

2. Add highlights to AV panel to add width.

3. Bottom flip-out adds width. Add Division C highlights to create width.

4. Side-swept fringe adds width at the temple area and creates a vertical line.

5. Long layer pieces should flip out. Add lightness to the ends.

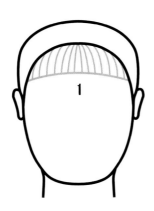

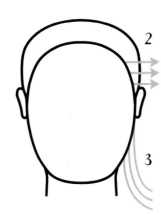

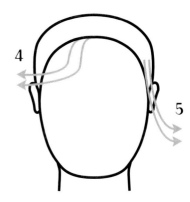

Diamond

1. Highlights in the ¼, ½, or ¾ HP area to add width to narrow forehead area.

2. Division AV panel needs to be left dark or colored one shade darker. Do not place highlights in the widest part of the face.

3. Highlight Division C at the bottom of the hairline to create width at the narrow chin.

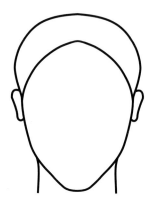

Narrow chin, forehead wide through the cheek area.

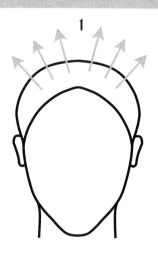

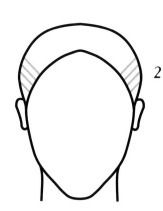

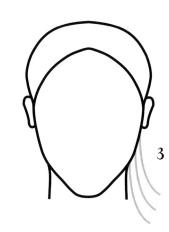

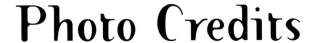

Photo Credits

We would like to thank Toshihiko Sawajiri for his beautiful photography. A professional photographer, Toshi has specialized in sports photography for the last twenty years. Beginning his career as a water-sports photographer, capturing events such as surfing, Jet-Skiing , and yachting, he then began focusing on a main stream sports for MLB, NBA, NFL, professional tennis, and many others. He has covered most of the major sporting events in the USA, including the Super Bowl, NBA Finals, US Open, and Masters Golf Tournament. Toshi was born and raised in Japan, and moved to the United States in 1984.

Thank you to each of Billy Yamaguchi's clients who were involved in this project. We appreciate your time and your willingness to allow us to show your beauty to the world through the pictures in this book.

Ally Crane	Heidi Meek	Martha Zilm
Amy Foster	Idolia Barbu	Mary Lou Fonzo
Anna Lee Cox	Jamie Morel	Megan Dempster
Anne Wibbelmann	Jean Faught	Mikella Polito
Ashlee Dana	Jennifer Roth	Mindy Maloon
Bailee Davis	Jessica Cooper	Nancy Clancy
Bernita E. Gray	Jocelyn C. Collis	Norma Fioretti
Brittany Elliott	Kanako Hamahira	Pam Mayer
Brittney McWethy	Katherine Anne Rocklin	Pamela Bermann
Chris Rennolds	Kathy Ikemire	Rebeca Elliott
Christine Burkhart	Kimberly Vonch	Sachi Yano
Dawn Dana	Kimberly Walters	Sammie Needham
Denise Aguiling	Laura Robin	Sara Bashor
Diana Smith	Leigh Ann Dunkle	Sara Peyton
Donna Barranco Fisher	Leslie Ferrell	Sarah Piring
Doreen Alvarado	Leslie McWethy	Sayaka Nagasawa
Elizabeth Thelander	Linda Wachold	Shandee Billings
Gail Smith	Lisa Munoz	Stephanie Gustafson
Gwendolyn Lauterbach	Lizzy Hare	Taeko Magallanes
Hayley Karch	Lois Fischman	Victoria Adam
Heather Harris	Lori White	

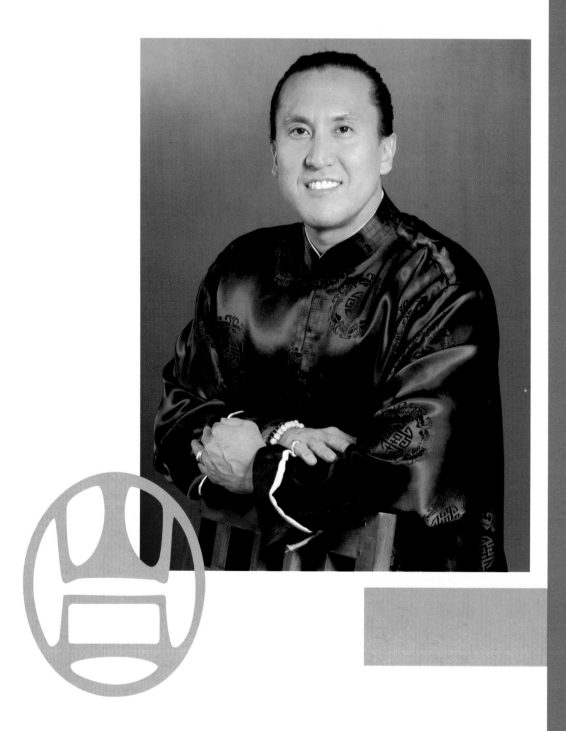

About the Author

BILLY YAMAGUCHI is president and co-owner of Yamaguchi International, which includes five California salon locations in Ventura, Spa La Quinta in La Quinta, La Costa Resort in San Diego, the St. Regis Spa and Century Plaza Hotel in Los Angeles, and several more under development in other states.

During his eighteen-year career, Billy has led seminars and workshops for beauty and skincare professionals throughout North America, Europe, Asia, South America, the Philippines, and South Africa.

He has been featured in *Vogue, W, Glamour, Town & Country,* and *BrideMagazine* as well as on ABC and CBS, the Style Network, Lifetime, *E! Entertainment, Ricki Lake,* and many others. His salons have served such celebrity clients as Jennifer Aniston, Lisa Kudrow, Courteney Cox Arquette, Julia Roberts, Mel Gibson, Drew Barrymore, Brooke Shields, Kate Moss, Phil Jackson, Ashley Judd, and *Queer Eye for the Straight Guy* star Carson Kressley.

More than ten years ago Billy began his study of Feng Shui and a quest to wed this philosophy to his training in the Western tradition of hair design. He soon discovered there was no existing method of integrating these disciplines and he devoted himself to combining the elements into an entirely innovative approach to beauty and harmony. Billy has brought the fundamentals of hair artistry and the Feng Shui principles as they are applied to beauty to a worldwide community of stylists. Closer to home, Billy established the Yamaguchi University where he, his wife, Melissa Chambers Yamaguchi, and Team Yamaguchi teach the Art of Feng Shui in Beauty. Billy has published *Yamaguchi Feng Shui: The Art & Science of Color Formulation* for salon professionals.

Yamaguchi Salon Locations

Yamaguchi Salon & Day Spa
1794 S. Victoria Ave, Ste 2A
Ventura, CA 93003
805-568-7909

Yamaguchi Salon @ Spa La Quinta
La Quinta Resort & CLub
49-499 Eisenhower Dr.
La Quinta, CA 92253
760-777-4888

Yamaguchi Salon @ St. Regis Spa
St. Regis Hotel
2055 Avenue of the Stars
Los Angeles, CA 90067
310-551-7577

Yamaguchi Salon @ Spa Mystique
Century Plaza Hotel
2025 Avenue of the Stars
Los Angeles, CA 90067
310-551-7577

Yamaguchi Salon @ La Costa
La Costa Resort
2100 Costa Del Mar Road
Carlsbad, CA 92009
460-438-0551

Please visit our website at www.yamaguchifengshui.com

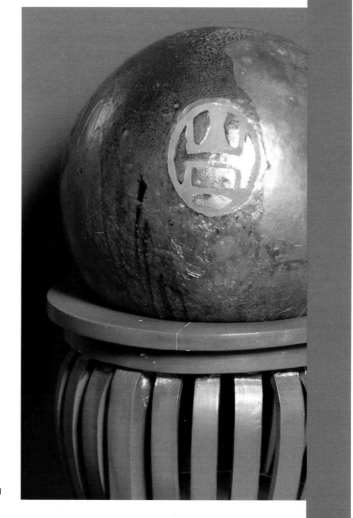

BOSTON PUBLIC LIBRARY

3 9999 05375 275 2

R